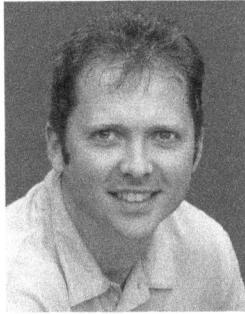

Andrew Cate is a personal trainer and online weight-loss coach. He writes for several magazines and websites, and can be heard regularly on radio sharing his passion for health, food and fitness. Many people have found success with his books *Throw Out Your Scales*, *Walk Off Weight*, *Lighten Up* and *The H-Factor Diet*.

The Fast Food Detox — ABC Books

The Tight Ar$e Diet — ABC Books

The H-Factor Diet — ABC Books

Lighten Up — ABC Books

Walk Off Weight — ABC Books

Throw Out Your Scales — ABC Books

Taste Testers for Weight Loss — Allen & Unwin

Gutbusters Low Fat Snacks and Sweets — Allen & Unwin

Slim, Trim and Tasty — JB Fairfax

Healthy Heart for Life

Lower your blood pressure and cholesterol in just 6 weeks

Andrew Cate

ABC
Books

The ABC 'Wave' device is a trademark of the
Australian Broadcasting Corporation and is used
under licence by HarperCollins*Publishers* Australia.

First published in 2012
by HarperCollins*Publishers* Australia Pty Limited
ABN 36 009 913 517
harpercollins.com.au

HarperCollins*Publishers*
Level 13, 201 Elizabeth Street, Sydney, NSW 2000, Australia
31 View Road, Glenfield, Auckland 0627, New Zealand
A 53, Sector 57, Noida, UP, India
77–85 Fulham Palace Road, London W6 8JB, United Kingdom
2 Bloor Street East, 20th floor, Toronto, Ontario M4W 1A8, Canada
10 East 53rd Street, New York NY 10022, USA

National Library of Australia Cataloguing-in-Publication data:

Cate, Andrew.
  Healthy heart for life / Andrew Cate.
  ISBN: 978 0 7333 2887 9 (pbk.)
  Heart – Diseases – Prevention.
616.1205

Cover design by Darren Holt, HarperCollins Design Studio
Cover Images by shutterstock.com
Typeset in Garth Graphic Regular by Yvonne Fillery

This book is dedicated to the memory of my two grandfathers, Rex Lackey and Jack Cate.

Contents

Introduction

Something had to be wrong. I was called in to see the headmaster in the middle of class. Being a studious 11-year-old who had never been sent to the headmaster's office before, it was a nervous walk. I wondered what I could possibly have done that was so bad. My homework was finished and I always completed my assignments on time. Maybe it was a good thing. Maybe I was in line for an award for outstanding service to the underrated sport of handball? Probably not.

When I arrived at the headmaster's office, my brother was there too, and we were told that our parents were about to pick us up at the front of the school. When I saw my mother's face I wished I was in trouble with the headmaster. Something was definitely wrong.

My wonderful grandfather had just died of a heart attack at the tender age of 67. It's the first time I can remember feeling totally empty. My life had been all fun, football and tadpoles up until then. I was desperately sad and there was nothing anyone could do or say to make me feel better. That feeling is something I'll never forget and, sadly, it's a feeling that was repeated several years later when my other grandfather died of lung cancer.

These events and feelings ultimately guided me down the path towards pursuing further studies in health science and human movement. I have also taken every opportunity to promote health and wellness as a personal trainer and a writer. If this book can help to prevent, reverse or delay heart disease in just one person, it will all be worth it. If this book helps to prevent or delay the suffering of friends and family who know someone with heart disease, it will all be worth it. I owe it to the memory of my grandfathers.

Heart disease has obviously had a significant impact on my life. It's probably had an impact on your life too, either directly or indirectly. Heart disease prevents millions of people from living a full life.

If you have ever been in any doubt about how serious a problem heart disease is, take a look at these alarming statistics.

- More people than ever are living with heart disease. It's estimated that one in four Australians over the age of 25 has high blood pressure.
- Six million Australians are thought to have high blood cholesterol.
- Heart disease is the leading cause of death globally, and more people die annually from heart disease than from any other cause.
- In industrialised countries, around one in two people will die

from heart and blood vessel disease. Many of these deaths are preventable.

- Heart disease kills five times more women than breast cancer.
- Every day, 150 Australians die from cardiovascular disease, and it's not just the elderly, with 8000 men and 3000 women under the age of 65 losing their life to heart disease each year.
- Billions of dollars are spent every year on medical devices and drugs to treat heart disease.
- More than 50 per cent of people who die suddenly of a heart attack had no signs or symptoms of heart disease.

Did you read all those statistics? Do you think that it won't happen to you? That's what my grandfather thought as well. Although a heart attack is sudden, it usually results from a process that takes many years to develop. What's more, heart disease is not an inevitable result of ageing — it's largely preventable.

Fortunately it's not all doom and gloom. Yes, I know that for all of us our time will be up one day, but it makes a lot of sense to make the journey as long-lasting and enjoyable as possible. And that's what this book is really all about. *Healthy Heart for Life* is designed to show you practical ways to modify your lifestyle to help you live a long and vibrant life. The tips in this book are easy to follow and are based on scientific research, which means they are proven to be effective.

And it's scientific research that helped to design the format of *Healthy Heart for Life*. You may have noticed the subtitle is 'The 6-week plan to lower your blood pressure and cholesterol naturally'. In 2005, the *Journal of the American Dietetic Association* reported on a study where people made a significant difference to their heart health within six weeks. After making some simple lifestyle changes, people experienced significant reductions in body fat, cholesterol levels and blood pressure. Doesn't that sound great? After just six weeks, these people were facing a future with a dramatic reduction in the risk of killer illnesses like heart disease, not to mention diabetes and even cancer. The lifestyle changes that took place in this groundbreaking study are the types of change I'll guide you through in this book.

Obviously, your heart health and therefore your quality and quantity of life will benefit most from lifestyle changes that are permanent. Make no mistake: this is not a diet or a fad that you can just start and stop if you want lasting changes to your health. It's great to know you can also achieve meaningful results in such a short space of time.

Healthy Heart for Life is about making one change each day over six weeks — all up, 42 days. Over the next six weeks, you'll discover how achievable it is to adopt a new perspective on lifestyle strategy. You'll see how a series of lifestyle practices will impact on your heart health and longevity.

These claims and strategies are based on peer-reviewed scientific research, which you'll see in the 'Science says' section of each of the 42 new practices. I've summarised over 200 scientific studies, whittling them down to the bare essentials. In other words, there's no scientific jargon or mumbo jumbo — just the plain facts that apply to your life now and in the future.

Finally, most new practices include a series of tips that show you what specific changes you can make to your lifestyle that day, and from that day onwards. You only need to adopt one new practice a day. Keep in mind that over the six-week program, those daily changes will snowball and there will be support for you along the way to keep you focused.

I appreciate you giving me the opportunity to boost your health. Let's enjoy the journey together. Read on, follow my tips and you will experience how a stronger heart will not only help you live longer but live better.

Be well,

Andrew Cate

Day 1

Identify your risk factors for heart disease

WHAT IS THE IMPACT ON YOUR HEALTH?

Your heart is a muscular pump supplying blood to your body through an extensive network of blood vessels, also known as your arteries and veins. Blood pumped by the heart supplies the muscles and tissues with the oxygen and nutrients needed for maintenance, growth and repair. It also carries away waste materials that are then filtered and processed for removal. The heart itself is a strong muscle. It will typically beat about once a second, every minute of your life, although it beats considerably faster during exercise and slower when you sleep. It's a pretty special little organ, and it has a strong influence on your health and wellbeing. The main underlying problem with heart disease is a gradual clogging of your blood vessels caused by fatty cholesterol deposits. This gradual build-up on the inside walls of the arteries narrows the passage that blood passes through, increasing blood pressure levels. This is known as atherosclerosis. Arterial plaque forms through a combination of free radical damage, formation of scar tissue, platelets, calcium, cholesterol and triglycerides, which are used in the blood vessel to heal the injury. It may also harden the arteries and make them less flexible, which is also known as atherosclerosis (although it may also be called arteriosclerosis, and these terms are often used interchangeably). High blood cholesterol and high blood pressure are two of the most significant risk factors for heart disease.

TAKE THE QUIZ TO HELP IDENTIFY YOUR RISK FACTORS

Knowledge is power, especially when it comes to heart disease because it can be prevented or successfully treated when detected early. The greatest risk factor for heart disease is not knowing what your individual risk factors are. Without knowing you are at risk, you won't have the opportunity to adjust your lifestyle to reduce your level of risk. The following quiz is designed to assess your personal areas of risk for heart disease, and help you develop a better understanding of the specific lifestyle factors you can modify to reduce your risk. Some of these factors (such as age and gender) are beyond your control, while others (such as diet and exercise) you can control.

UNCONTROLLABLE RISK FACTORS

1. What is your gender?

   a. Female

   b. Male

   Score 1 point for a, and 2 points for b.

   > Men are at an increased risk of heart disease but heart disease is still a significant issue for women, especially after menopause.

2. How old are you?

   a. Under 40

   b. 40–50

   c. Over 50

   Score 1 point for a, 2 points for b, and 3 points for c.

   > As you age, your risk of suffering heart disease increases. Pay careful attention to the risk factors you can control to offset this.

3. What is your family history of heart disease?

   a. No premature heart disease before the age of 55

   b. Don't know

   c. Heart disease in the family before age 55

   Score 1 point for a, 2 points for b, and 3 points for c.

If you have a family history of heart disease, this can increase your level of risk. Instead of this being an excuse to say 'Woe is me,' it's really an even better reason to pay careful attention to the risk factors that are within your control.

CONTROLLABLE RISK FACTORS

4. What is your smoking status?

    a. Non-smoker

    b. 15 or less cigarettes per day

    c. Over 15 cigarettes per day

    Score 1 point for a, 2 points for b, and 3 points for c.

    Smoking is associated with significant levels of premature death. It's never too late to give up, as you'll see on Day 18.

5. What was your blood pressure when tested in the past two years?

    a. Low or normal (<120/<80)

    b. Slightly elevated or you don't know your blood pressure (120–160/81–99)

    c. High or you are on medication to reduce your blood pressure (160+/100+)

    Score 1 point for a, 2 points for b, and 3 points for c.

High blood pressure is one of the most significant risk factors for heart disease. You can learn more about it on pages 21–26.

6. What was your blood cholesterol level when tested in the past two years?
    a. Low or below 5.5 mmol/litre
    b. Average, on 5.5 mmol/litre, or you don't know your cholesterol level
    c. High, over 5.5 mmol/litre, or you are on medication to reduce your cholesterol level

    Score 1 point for a, 2 points for b, and 3 points for c.

Cholesterol deposits contribute to atherosclerosis, which narrows and hardens your arteries. There are different types of cholesterol that you will learn more about on Day 2.

7. How would you describe your weight?
    a. Normal, healthy weight
    b. Overweight or underweight
    c. Very overweight or obese

    Score 1 point for a, 2 points for b, and 3 points for c.

Excess body fat is associated with high blood pressure and increased levels of blood fats that can make life difficult for your heart. While Day 4 focuses specifically on losing body fat, many of the healthy lifestyle strategies outlined throughout *Healthy Heart for Life* will help you to manage your weight.

8. How much exercise do you undertake each week?

    a. More than 5 hours per week

    b. 1–5 hours per week

    c. Less than 1 hour per week

    Score 1 point for a, 2 points for b, and 3 points for c.

Inactivity ranks alongside smoking and high blood pressure as a major risk factor for heart disease. You will learn more on how to boost your activity levels on Days 6, 16 and 31.

9. How would you describe your diet?

    a. Healthy — high in vegetables and fibre, low in fat, salt and sugar

    b. OK — sometimes healthy

    c. Poor — high in fat, fast food and sugar

    Score 1 point for a, 2 points for b, and 3 points for c.

Diet is one of the key modifiable risk factors for heart disease. Several sections throughout this book focus on what foods to eat more of and what to eat less of.

10. What is your diabetes status?
    a. You are not a diabetic and there is no history of diabetes in your family
    b. You are not a diabetic but there is a history of diabetes in your family
    c. You are a diabetic

    Score 1 point for a, 2 points for b, and 3 points for c.

    Diabetics face a heightened risk of heart disease, although that risk can be reduced by a healthy lifestyle that keeps a tight control over blood sugar levels. Day 30 looks at some key food strategies to control your blood sugar levels.

11. How would you describe your stress levels and attitude to life?
    a. Easy-going and content
    b. Sometimes hurried and intolerant
    c. Often hurried and aggressive

    Score 1 point for a, 2 points for b, and 3 points for c.

Stress has a big impact on your cardiovascular health. Days 15 and 36 look at how to manage stress and how to relax more to compensate for its harmful effects.

12. How much alcohol do you drink?
    a. I don't drink alcohol
    b. I drink 1–2 (women) or 2–3 (men) glasses a day and have two to four alcohol-free days a week
    c. I binge drink, drink quickly or drink more than is described in point b

    Score 1 point for a, 1 point for b, and 3 points for c.

Drinking too much alcohol can raise blood pressure and triglycerides, and contribute to the storage of excess body fat. Day 14 offers a series of tips on how to drink in moderation, which can actually boost your heart health.

Now, add up the total score and check your result with the corresponding score levels below to determine your level of risk for heart disease.

Use your answers to the quiz to identify specific controllable risk factors you can work on to lower your risk. You might like to focus on the relevant chapters for each of the controllable risk factors you identify.

SCORE 12–17

Your risk of heart disease is low. Stick with your healthy lifestyle habits, making sure you exercise regularly and that your weight, blood pressure and cholesterol levels are low.

SCORE 18–26

Your risk of heart disease is moderate. While some of the factors increasing your risk of heart disease may be beyond your control, you could still focus more on exercise and a healthy diet to keep down your weight, blood pressure and cholesterol levels.

SCORE 27–35

Your risk of heart disease is high. It is vital that you focus on the key lifestyle factors that you can control and improve upon such as exercise, stress management, weight, blood pressure and cholesterol.

Day 2

Lower your bad cholesterol and increase the good

WHAT IS THE IMPACT ON YOUR HEALTH?

Cholesterol is a fatty substance found in the blood that multitasks. It is a component in every cell in your body, helping to form cell membranes and hormones, and is an essential ingredient in bile acids that help you to digest dietary fat. The liver uses fats and glucose to produce cholesterol, making all the cholesterol your body needs to perform these important functions. However, some people produce more cholesterol than their body needs, especially when the diet contains saturated and trans fats. Eating cholesterol-rich foods — which are all animal products, with prawns, eggs and offal being particularly high in cholesterol — has a minimal effect on raising your blood cholesterol levels compared to saturated and trans fats. Excess body fat and hereditary factors can also elevate cholesterol levels. Because fat and watery blood don't mix well, cholesterol is transported around your bloodstream by lipoproteins. The type of lipoprotein that cholesterol attaches to and the degree to which it is oxidised (depending on your antioxidant intake) will determine the health risks involved. The composition of these lipoproteins includes differing proportions of protein, cholesterol and other fats (triglycerides). The three most common forms of lipoproteins are:

- **Low-density lipoprotein or LDL** — This is the 'bad' type of cholesterol that is thought to deposit plaque on your artery walls, narrowing your blood vessels. If there is a reduction in the delivery of blood and oxygen to the heart, chest pain (angina) can occur. If a clot or blockage occurs in the heart or brain that stops the flow of blood completely, a heart attack or stroke can occur.

- **High-density lipoprotein or HDL** — This is often referred to as the 'good' cholesterol because it carries cholesterol and other fats away from the arteries and back to the liver for disposal. It helps to prevent the build-up of arterial plaque and can help to prevent heart disease.

- **Very low-density lipoprotein or VLDL** — This lesser known type of cholesterol mainly carries blood fats (triglycerides) from the liver and can be converted into LDL. It also contributes to cholesterol build-up in your blood vessels and increases the risk of heart disease.

WHAT SHOULD YOUR CHOLESTEROL LEVEL BE?

The sum of your three types of cholesterol usually combines to make up your total cholesterol levels, and it's recommended that your total cholesterol levels be less than 5.5 mmol/litre. Coronary heart disease is rare in individuals with a blood cholesterol level below 4.5 mmol/litre. More specifically, the suggested target levels that make up your total cholesterol are:

- LDL-cholesterol <2.0 mmol/litre
- HDL-cholesterol >1.0 mmol/litre
- VDL-(triglycerides) <1.5 mmol/litre

WHAT IS THE LDL TO HDL RATIO?

Because HDL makes up a small portion of your cholesterol levels, total cholesterol is generally used as a measure of heart risk. Total cholesterol is also cheap and easy to measure. However, there's a strong argument that the proportion of HDL to LDL is a more reliable indicator of heart disease risk. A doctor might be inclined to look at your HDL to LDL ratio if your total cholesterol is high. You can calculate your HDL to LDL cholesterol ratio (HDL/LDL) by dividing your HDL cholesterol level by your LDL cholesterol value. For example, if your HDL cholesterol is 0.8 mmol/litre, and your LDL is 2.4mmol/litre, then your ratio of HDL to LDL is 0.33. Ideally, your HDL to LDL ratio should be above 0.3. Women generally have a higher ratio of HDL to LDL compared to men, which reduces their risk of heart disease. It's thought that oestrogen may be involved in elevating HDL levels and protecting women's health because this effect is lost once a woman reaches menopause and oestrogen levels diminish. People who exercise regularly are also more likely to have high HDL to LDL levels because of the favourable effects of physical activity, which is known to increase HDL cholesterol levels and reduce LDL cholesterol levels.

THE CHOLESTEROL DEBATE

There's an argument that the conventional three-part cholesterol measurement is a poor predictor of heart disease risk. Technically, there are other lesser-known types of cholesterol that also impact on your risk of heart disease, such as apolipoprotein(a) and apolipoprotein(b). According to research in the medical journal *The Lancet*, they have a better predictive power than HDL and LDL cholesterol but more work needs to be done to help standardise testing methods. We will probably hear more about them in the future.

For the purposes of this book, and more importantly boosting your heart health and wellness, I've tried to keep things simple (and effective). Personally, I think cholesterol is a useful measure (especially your HDL to LDL ratio) as long as you recognise that it is one of many factors that determine your heart disease risk.

Ultimately, the lifestyle changes I will guide you through will address all the major risk factors of heart disease, and many of these will help improve your balance of good and bad cholesterol. This includes foods to eat more of (garlic, vegetables, high-fibre grain foods and seafood), and foods to eat less of (sugar, trans fats and saturated fats).

SCIENCE SAYS

Low 'good' cholesterol is dangerous — According to the *Archives of Internal Medicine*, low levels of 'good' cholesterol, rather than high levels of 'bad' cholesterol, are associated with an increased risk of death from heart disease and stroke in older people. This echoes data from a study published in the *Annals of Internal Medicine* that found when patients' HDL was increased, coronary plaques stopped progressing, even showing signs of regression. The risk of heart events also went down by 52 per cent.

Eggs are OK in moderation — According to the Heart Foundation it's OK to eat up to six eggs each week as part of a healthy balanced diet. Eggs contain omega-3 fats plus a number of vitamins and minerals. They also contain around 5 grams of fat but most of this is the 'good' unsaturated fat that you need to be healthy. There is only about 1.5 grams of saturated fat and eggs contain no trans fat. The dietary cholesterol in eggs has only a small effect on LDL cholesterol, although some people are more sensitive to the dietary cholesterol in eggs than others. Of more concern is the much greater impact that saturated and trans fats have on LDL cholesterol, especially in the foods that accompany eggs such as bacon, sausages and hash browns.

Exercise boosts 'good' cholesterol — A study reported in the journal *Arteriosclerosis, Thrombosis, and Vascular Biology* has shown that regular endurance exercise can increase the levels of 'good' cholesterol. The men in this study exercised for 50 minutes a day, three times a week; they also lost body fat. According to the researchers, the intensity of the exercise was less important than the duration.

Day 3

Lower your blood pressure or maintain it at a healthy level

WHAT IS THE IMPACT ON YOUR HEALTH?

Blood pressure is a measure of the force of your blood pushing against the walls of your arteries as it is being pumped around your body by your heart. The flow and pressure of blood through your blood vessels results in two numbers, which are labelled:

- **Systolic pressure** — Pressure rises with each beat of your heart and this top or higher number is known as systolic pressure.
- **Diastolic pressure** — When the heart relaxes and refills, pressure is reduced and this lower reading is known as the diastolic pressure.

WHAT IS A HEALTHY BLOOD PRESSURE READING?

Blood pressure is measured using a sphygmomanometer, where a cuff is inflated around the upper arm to get a reading of the blood inside the arteries. This results in a reading such as 120/80 mmHg (millimetres of mercury), which is expressed as '120 over 80'. Blood pressure readings vary among individuals, and throughout the day, so there is no perfect number. For some people the stress of being tested by their doctor is enough to raise blood pressure to artificially high levels and is known as 'white coat hypertension'. The following table offers some guidelines for adults.

Category	Blood Pressure Level (mmHg) Systolic	Blood Pressure Level (mmHg) Diastolic
Normal	Less than 120	Less than 80
Pre-hypertension	120–139	80–89
Borderline high blood pressure	140–159	90–99
High, requires attention	160–179	100–109
Very high	180 and above	110 and above

WHAT CAUSES HIGH BLOOD PRESSURE?

A number of factors increase blood pressure such as excess body fat, physical inactivity and too much salt and alcohol in your diet. When the blood vessels become thinner or more rigid, the heart has to work harder to transport blood throughout your body. This increases the level of pressure in the pipes and tubes, further damaging the lining of your arteries. This increases your risk of getting heart disease, stroke and kidney disease. According to research, a high systolic reading is more of a concern than a high diastolic reading because a high systolic reading is a better predictor of risk for a heart attack.

High blood pressure (or hypertension) is also known as the 'silent killer' because you can't feel it. That's why it's important to know your blood pressure so that you can take steps to control it.

Blood pressure medication is one of Australia's largest prescription drug markets yet lifestyle changes can prevent, eliminate or reduce the amount of drugs needed to treat hypertension. While it's important that your doctor decides what treatment is most appropriate for you, there are lifestyle measures you can adopt which can make a difference and reduce your risk of suffering from high blood pressure.

WHO IS AT RISK OF DEVELOPING HIGH BLOOD PRESSURE?

It's thought that around one in four people above the age of 25 suffer from high blood pressure. There are three main factors that place people at a higher risk of developing hypertension, including:

- **People over 35 years of age** — Blood pressure increases with age, so the older you get, the greater your chance of developing high blood pressure. Men often develop hypertension between 35 and 55 years of age, while women tend to develop it after menopause.

- **People with a family history** — If someone in your immediate family has high blood pressure you have an increased tendency to develop the condition. If you have a family history of high blood pressure, pay extra attention to the lifestyle factors you can control.

- **People with an unhealthy lifestyle** — Our lives and our behaviour have a huge bearing on blood pressure. Lifestyle factors that increase the risk of heart disease, such as poor diet or inactivity, can have an impact from an early age. Continue following the *Healthy Heart for Life* six-week plan to give you a better understanding of the lifestyle behaviours that increase your risk of developing hypertension and, most importantly, what you can do to reduce your risk.

SCIENCE SAYS

Lifestyle changes alone can lower blood pressure — A report published in the *Journal of the American Medical Association* has shown that for an average person with poor lifestyle habits, a combination of lifestyle changes can reduce high blood pressure without drugs. The changes included 180 minutes of moderately intense exercise per week, a reduced-fat diet featuring plenty of fruits and vegetables, weight loss of at least 7 kilograms, reduced salt intake and limiting alcoholic beverages to one serve per day for women and two for men.

Pre-hypertension is still a danger — According to findings published in the *New England Journal of Medicine*, people with blood pressure levels that tend to be slightly elevated but fall within what are considered normal ranges are still at an increased risk of suffering from heart disease. Pre-hypertension, or high-normal for the purposes of this 10-year study, was classified as a systolic pressure of 130 to 139 or a diastolic pressure of 85 to 89. Women with high-normal blood pressure had a 2.5 times greater risk of heart disease compared to those with normal blood pressure, while men with high-normal values had 1.6 times greater risk of heart disease.

Blood pressure warning for the obese — A study in the journal *Hypertension* has found that as weight increases, so do blood pressure levels. Obese people were often found to have increased blood pressure levels compared to normal-weight individuals. It was also discovered that obese people may not experience the night-time drop in blood pressure that occurs in normal-weight individuals, a phenomenon that could result in damage to the heart.

Prevention is better than medication — Lifestyle guidelines published in the *Journal of the American Medical Association* on how to lower blood pressure stress the importance of prevention of hypertension. According to the researchers, once someone develops high blood pressure they are often on medication for life. This is not only expensive but reduces quality of life. Ultimately, it's better not to develop hypertension in the first place. The researchers recommend keeping trim, exercising, cutting back on saturated fats, limiting alcohol and salt, and eating plenty of fruits and vegetables.

Home blood pressure monitoring can be helpful — The American Heart Association has issued its support for home monitoring as part of an overall management plan for high blood pressure. While still working with a doctor, home monitoring is a convenient way for tracking blood pressure over long periods of time, and it may encourage people to maintain better blood pressure control by being aware of any changes. Home monitoring may be particularly helpful for people with white coat hypertension — people whose blood pressure jumps as soon as they're face to face with a doctor.

Day 4

Lose and/or maintain a healthy level of body fat (especially around the tummy)

WHAT IS THE IMPACT ON YOUR HEALTH?

Excess body fat puts considerable stress on your heart. It's been estimated that for every additional kilogram of body fat you carry, the body has to grow a few extra kilometres of new blood vessels and small arteries. Excess body fat is closely linked with high blood pressure, high blood cholesterol and diabetes, and is a known risk factor for heart disease. What's more, it's not just what you weigh but where you carry your weight that also determines your level of risk. Fat stored in and around the tummy and internal organs (resulting in a pot belly or apple shape) makes you more prone to heart problems and diabetes.

Fat stored internally is called 'visceral fat' and it has even stronger links with type 2 diabetes, heart disease and strokes than general body fat. You can have visceral fat even if you're thin. This deep abdominal fat is thought to be more metabolically active (more readily released into the bloodstream), unlike the stubborn fat stored on the buttocks and thighs. Researchers suspect one of the main reasons why men are more susceptible to heart disease is because they tend to store fat around the mid-section. For all these reasons, losing excess body fat is one of the most important lifestyle strategies you can adopt to reduce your risk of heart disease.

SCIENCE SAYS

Overweight people suffer heart attacks earlier — A study reported in the journal *Clinical Cardiology* showed that overweight people were more likely to experience a heart attack at a younger age compared to people of normal weight. The study found that, on average, normal-weight heart attack victims experienced a heart attack 3.6 years later than overweight adults, and 8.2 years after obese subjects.

Waist management — Research published in the *British Medical Journal* has proven that a waist circumference of more than 94 centimetres in men and 80 centimetres in women indicates a person is nearly twice as likely to have one or more risk factors for heart disease compared to those with smaller waists. A waist circumference of more than 100 centimetres in men and 90 centimetres in women indicates an unhealthy level of body fat that requires a reduction in girth otherwise health problems are highly likely to occur.

Waist circumference predicts heart disease risk — According to the *American Journal of Clinical Nutrition,* waist circumference is a better indicator of your risk for heart disease than body mass index (BMI or weight in relation to height). Abdominal fat was a stronger measure of cholesterol levels, blood pressure and blood glucose levels. A waist measurement above 101 centimetres in men and 94 centimetres in women corresponds to the highest cardiovascular disease risk.

Your gut could be making you fat — A study reported in the journal of the Federation of American Societies for Experimental Biology has suggested that the extra fat you carry around the belly could increase hunger levels, triggering further weight gain. The study found that a potent hunger hormone called Neuropeptide Y (NPY) is reproduced by abdominal fatty tissue. The concern is that a vicious cycle could develop where NPY from excess body fat causes you to eat more and gain even more fat around your middle.

Lose a little, gain a lot — According to a study published in the journal *Circulation,* obese people who lose even a small amount of weight may significantly reduce their chance of heart disease. Weight loss results in a reduction in the number of proteins known as cytokines, which are thought to cause inflammation that contributes to formation of fat deposits in arteries. Subjects who lost an average of 9 kilograms experienced a return to a safe level of cytokines in the blood.

Obesity lops off lifespan — A study published in the *Journal of the American Medical Association* has reported that obesity is a well-known risk factor for heart disease and is a leading cause of premature death. According to researchers, it can cut a person's lifespan by between 10 and 20 years.

Yo-yo diet danger — A study documented in the *Journal of the American College of Cardiology* found that individuals who constantly lose weight and then put it back on again may develop lower levels of HDL (good) cholesterol, putting them at increased risk of heart disease. The researchers found that women who lost at least 4 kilograms three or more times in their life had 7 per cent lower HDL cholesterol than women who maintained a stable weight. This may be particularly important for women because HDL cholesterol appears to be a better predictor of heart disease in women than in men.

Weight loss lowers blood pressure — According to the medical journal *Hypertension*, reducing body fat levels should be a major focus in the treatment of high blood pressure. A review of 25 trials found that the more weight people lost, the more their blood pressure was reduced.

Exercise trims tummy fat and lessens heart risk — Research reported in the *Journal of the American Medical Association* found that regular exercise helps trim tummy fat and lower the risk of heart disease. Post-menopausal women who began an exercise program of brisk walking or cycling for 45 minutes on five days a week lowered their levels of abdominal fat by about 6 per cent over 12 months. The researchers found that losing 1 kilogram of weight was associated with a 1 per cent reduction in cholesterol, and a 2 per cent reduction in triglycerides.

PRACTICAL TIPS ON HOW TO LOSE OR MAINTAIN A HEALTHY LEVEL OF BODY FAT

In its most basic form, weight control is about kilojoules in versus kilojoules out. Burn off more kilojoules than you take in and you will lose excess body fat. But there are a number of factors within this equation that need to be considered, and their importance will vary among different people. The following tips are designed to help reduce your kilojoule intake, increase your kilojoule expenditure and manage the other factors that help control body fat.

- Determine if you need to lose body fat. Because of the higher health risks associated with abdominal fat, waist circumference is a better indicator of the need to reduce body fat than total body weight. The following table can help assess your level of risk, measuring your waist at the belly button.

Health risk	Low	Medium	High
WOMEN Waist circumference	less than 80 cm	80 cm–88 cm	88 cm or more
MEN Waist circumference	less than 94 cm	94 cm–102 cm	102 cm or more

- Even if your waist measurement is currently healthy, there is no guarantee that it will remain so. Preventing weight gain is an important strategy to avoid the health problems associated with excess body fat. Continue to monitor your body fat levels and prevent a gradual creeping on of kilograms. Monitor your waist circumference once every month; this allows you to detect changes early and be proactive by adjusting your lifestyle accordingly. Because adults tend to gain weight during middle age, staying the same weight is an achievement worth striving for and celebrating. And of course many of people lose weight successfully but then fail to keep it off or gain even more weight afterwards. It's not just preventing weight gain that's important, but also preventing weight re-gain as well.

- If there is heart disease in your family, or if either of your parents are overweight, pay extra attention to keeping your levels of body fat at a healthy level. There are a number of strategies you can employ to help cut back on your kilojoule intake in a heart healthy way to maximise weight loss, and many of these are discussed throughout *Healthy Heart for Life*. Some examples include moderating your fat and sugar intake, eating plenty of legumes, vegetables and fibre, drinking plenty of water instead of kilojoule-laden drinks and watching your portion sizes.

- To boost your expenditure of kilojoules for weight management, engage in a regular program of physical activity. See Days 6, 16 and 31 for detailed information on how to exercise safely and effectively.

- Don't hesitate to team up with a friend or health professional in order to to be successful at losing weight. Whether it's a doctor, nutritionist, personal trainer or work colleague, it helps to have continual long-term support. Regular contact with a health professional can help provide motivation and up-to-date information. The internet is a great way to find extra information, advice and support. If you'd like to subscribe to my free weekly email newsletter, check the details at the back of this book.

Day 5

Reduce the level of inflammation in your body

WHAT IS THE IMPACT ON YOUR HEALTH?

We are increasing our understanding of the role inflammation plays in the development of a number of diseases, including heart disease. Inflammation is your body's response to injury or trauma such as a cut, bruise, bacteria or virus. It is the body's defensive response as it repairs damage and may result in heat, redness or tenderness.

On a cellular level, lifestyle-related factors like excess body fat, stress, smoking, pollution, inadequate sleep and inactivity are also thought to trigger a type of chronic, low-grade inflammation (called 'metaflammation') that affects the lining of the blood vessels. The processes that help form a scar after a cut are similar to the plaque that forms in your arteries from chronic metaflammation. It's also thought to thicken the blood and trigger the formation of blood clots, increasing the risk of high blood pressure and heart attacks.

Metaflammation can be measured in the body by checking the level of a substance known as C-reactive protein (CRP). Unlike total cholesterol, CRP seems to be a very good indicator for heart disease. It's possible you can have healthy cholesterol levels but higher levels of CRP. A number of the healthy lifestyle changes discussed further on have an anti-inflammatory effect and help to prevent metaflammation.

SCIENCE SAYS

Inflammation triggers many diseases — According to a study reported in the journal *Neuroimmunomodulation*, inflammation is the link between lifestyle and many chronic diseases. Some of those diseases include heart disease, diabetes, visceral-type obesity, autoimmunity, metabolic syndrome and major depression. Research has shown that individuals whose arteries had narrowed from a build-up of plaque had significantly higher CRP levels than individuals with no arterial narrowing.

Exercise cuts inflammation — A study reported in the *Journal of Arteriosclerosis, Thrombosis, and Vascular Biology* has shown that people who are physically fit tend to have lower levels of a CRP, a marker of body-wide inflammation. The fitter the subjects, the lower their levels of CRP, with those who were classified as 'most fit' being 83 per cent less likely to have high CRPs than the least fit men. According to the researchers, the most dramatic improvements came to those able to get out of the lowest fitness group and become moderately in shape from walking for 30 minutes for five days a week (even if the 30 minutes was accumulated in bits and pieces). This is another demonstration of why exercise helps reduce a person's risk of heart disease and a host of other cardiovascular problems.

Keeping inflammation in check — *The Lancet* reported that people who drank moderately (classed as a drink or two per day, or five to seven a week) had significantly lower levels of CRP compared with non-drinkers and heavy drinkers. According to the researchers, inflammation is known to trigger gout and atherosclerosis and it is believed to play a role in heart disease and some cancers.

Fatty fish prevents inflammation — The *American Journal of Cardiology* reported on a study that found that a diet rich in fatty fish such as salmon and mackerel can protect the heart and blood vessels by reducing inflammation, which is thought to contribute to the build-up of plaque inside arteries. Subjects with the highest cell levels of docosahexaenoic acid (DHA), a type of omega-3 fatty acid found in fish such as salmon and mackerel, had lower levels of CRP in their blood. According to the researchers, omega-3 fatty acids may protect against inflammation by inhibiting the formation of inflammation-promoting proteins.

- TV time increases inflammation — Research published in the *Journal of the American College of Cardiology* found CRP was approximately two times higher in people spending more than four hours of screen time per day compared to those spending less than two hours a day. They claimed that prolonged sitting may place someone at greater risk of a cardiac event and that CRP, a well-established marker of low-grade inflammation, may help explain the link.

PRACTICAL TIPS TO REDUCE THE LEVEL OF INFLAMMATION IN YOUR BODY

- Be aware of, and take steps to avoid, the lifestyle triggers of metaflammation such as excess body fat; the consumption of saturated fats, trans fats, high glycaemic index (GI) foods, fructose, excessive salt, excessive alcohol and fast foods; stress; smoking; air pollution; inadequate sleep; inactivity and excessive exercise.
- Be aware of, and take steps to include in your lifestyle, anti-inflammatory stimuli such as fruits, vegetables, nuts, fish, green tea, garlic, herbs and spices, olive oil and dark chocolate and opt for low GI foods, a high-fibre diet, and moderate alcohol intake, Mediterranean diet, physical, regular activity and, if you are a smoker, stop smoking.
- You can actually have a blood test for CRP, which allows you to screen for this hidden metaflammation, helping you to develop a better understanding of your health. A CRP level under 1 milligram per litre of blood means you have a

low risk of cardiovascular disease, while 1 to 3 milligrams means your risk is intermediate, and more than 3 milligrams is considered high risk.

- Antioxidants act as a protecting agent against metaflammation. See Day 24 on how to boost your intake.
- Take steps to boost your immune system and build up your resistance to metaflammation. An overall healthy diet will help but some foods have unique anti-inflammatory properties. These foods include:
  - ✦ Blueberries — Packed with vitamins C, E and disease-fighting antioxidants.
  - ✦ Broccoli — A good source of vitamins A, C and folate and is also rich in phytochemicals (plant compounds that have protective properties).
  - ✦ Spinach — High in iron and antioxidants.
  - ✦ Green tea — Rich in antioxidants, which prevent cell damage from oxidation. It also promotes the secretion of interferon, which has virus-fighting properties. See Day 34 for more information on green tea.
  - ✦ Garlic — Stimulates the multiplication of infection-fighting white blood cells and also contains the phytochemical allicin, which has anti-bacterial properties. See Day 26 for more information on garlic.
  - ✦ Cold water fish — The omega-3 fats in cold water fish (salmon, tuna) create high blood levels of flu-fighting T cells and interferon.
  - ✦ Soy products — Contain protein and a wide variety of nutrients. Soy products are also rich in isoflavanoids,

which help to balance your hormone and cholesterol levels.

✦ Pumpkin — High in carotenoids and B group vitamins.

✦ Water — Drink six to eight glasses a day to stay well hydrated, which keeps the susceptible mucus membranes in your upper respiratory tract moist and resistant to infection.

If you struggle to eat a high-nutrient diet, consider supplementing your diet with vitamin C, vitamin E, carotene, selenium, zinc and omega-3 fats, which will ensure your immune system has all the building blocks it needs to fight inflammation.

Day 6

Include some planned physical activity in your day

WHAT IS THE IMPACT ON YOUR HEALTH?

Like all muscles the heart becomes stronger from regular exercise, helping it to deliver blood more efficiently throughout the body. It's been said that if exercise was a drug, it would be the most heavily prescribed treatment in the world. That's because exercise, or physical activity, offers a range of significant health benefits to your heart, including:

- lowers blood pressure
- reduces LDL (bad) cholesterol
- increases HDL (good) cholesterol
- lowers blood fats (triglycerides)
- lowers resting heart rate
- helps reduce excess body fat

- helps to maintain a healthy level of body fat
- improves control over blood sugar levels, and reduces need for insulin
- improves quality of sleep
- improves management of stress.

Moderate exercise also helps to boost your immune system and reduce inflammation, contributing to an increase in the circulation of antibodies called macrophages (the cells that attack bacteria). By contrast, excessive exercise without adequate recovery time can weaken your immune system and increase your susceptibility to illness.

SCIENCE SAYS

Exercise burns abdominal fat — Research published in the *Journal of Applied Physiology* has shown that there is a dose-response relationship between exercise amount and the removal of existing stores of abdominal fat. The more exercise you do the more likely you are to lose abdominal fat.

Exercise acts like a heart disease drug — According to an issue of *Circulation Research*, exercise can act like a drug on the blood vessels but without the side effects. Exercise was found to protect the blood vessels by stimulating an anti-inflammatory response from the increased blood flow generated by activity.

Exercise lowers inflammation — A report to the American College of Cardiology showed that regular exercise may help reduce blood levels of C-reactive protein (CRP), which is linked to inflammation and increased heart disease risk. The study of nearly 3000 adults found that those who got the most exercise had the lowest levels and this was seen in all groups, including smokers, non-smokers and those with and without heart disease.

Activity reduces stroke risk — The journal *Stroke* has reported on a study where moderate and high levels of physical activity helped to reduce the risk of having a stroke. Individuals with high levels of activity had a 27 per cent lower risk of stroke or death compared with subjects with low activity levels. According to the researchers, it is now established beyond reasonable doubt that high-level physical activity can be strongly recommended for the prevention of stroke.

Exercise slows atherosclerosis — Findings reported in the *American Journal of Medicine* demonstrate that physical activity slows the build-up of plaque in the arteries and the more vigorous the activity, the better. Subjects who engaged in vigorous aerobic activity at least 3.5 times per week showed three times less plaque thickening over a three-year period compared to sedentary subjects.

Drugs work better with exercise — The *Journal of the American College of Cardiology* has found that for reducing the risk of heart attack and other complications of heart disease, cholesterol-lowering drugs are good. However, they are more effective when combined with diet and exercise. Subjects exercised for at least half an hour four to five days a week and stuck to a diet in which 10 per cent or less of kilojoules came from fat.

Exercise improves cholesterol ratio — An in-depth study published in the *New England Journal of Medicine* has found that exercise helped to lower LDL cholesterol and raise HDL cholesterol. The more exercise the subjects did, the greater the improvement in cholesterol profile. Subjects in this study cycled, walked and ran, and underwent an initial period of two to three months during which the amount and intensity of exercise were gradually increased, followed by six months at the appropriate exercise prescription. The researchers also noted that even in subjects who had minimal changes in weight, there were still broad beneficial effects on the HDL to LDL ratio. It appears that even if you don't seem to be losing weight, exercise is still doing you good.

PRACTICAL TIPS ON HOW TO INCLUDE PLANNED PHYSICAL ACTIVITY IN YOUR DAY

* There are some circumstances when it's advisable to see a doctor before starting a new exercise program. Consult a doctor if you are aged 55 years or older; have a family history of heart disease; have had a previous heart attack or stroke; are very overweight; are a heavy smoker; have a medical condition such as diabetes, asthma, arthritis or high blood pressure; if you are taking prescribed medication; or if you have any doubts about your health.
* Take extra care during the early stages of your new

exercise program if you have a history of heart disease, if you are taking medication for blood pressure or cholesterol or if you have suffered a heart attack in the past. Your doctor or heart specialist will generally make recommendations for your exercise program based on your condition.

- Start any new program of exercise at a slow and steady pace, building up your duration over six to eight weeks. Be sure to always warm up and cool down. See an exercise specialist if you have any doubts.
- Choose a type of exercise that is rhythmic and continuous such as walking, jogging, swimming, cycling or rowing.
- Aim to exercise between three and five times each week, building up your duration to 20 to 40 minutes depending on your age and general level of phyiscal activity.
- Walking is often recommended as an easy way to begin a physical activity program because it does not require special facilities or equipment other than well-made, comfortable shoes and a safe place to walk.
- If you walk at night, be safe. Wear light-coloured or reflective clothing, walk facing oncoming traffic, walk in well-lit, populated areas and try to use a footpath. If you have any concerns, walk with a friend or partner.
- If you are wearing a radio or portable music player, keep the volume at a level where you can still hear car noise.
- It is vital that you find an activity that you enjoy and are likely to stick with over the long term. Try to vary the location, time of day, intensity and duration of your

exercise. This helps to keep your mind fresh and prevents boredom.

- Look for ways to progress after a few months as you get fitter. This may involve exercising for longer or more often or at a higher intensity. Set out a special personal best course over a given distance and try to beat your best time every week or two. You can even use gadgets like a heart rate monitor or pedometer to give you feedback.

- Once you have developed a reasonable foundation of fitness, a useful guide to your intensity during exercise is that you should be able to hear your breath. You don't want to be gasping for air but you should be able to hear yourself breathing.

- As your fitness improves you can try adding sporting activities such as touch football, tennis, squash, basketball and volleyball. While not ideal as your only form of exercise, sports can add a fun, social element and are a great complement to your exercise routine.

- While lack of time is a major excuse people use to avoid exercise, any time invested in movement will bring healthy returns. If you struggle for time or motivation, try to make an exercise appointment with yourself or find a training partner to exercise with.

- If you feel any pain, discomfort or dizziness during exercise, stop immediately. Don't try to push through it. 'No pain, no gain' is an irrelevant and misleading statement when it comes to exercise for cardiovascular health. Pain is a warning sign to stop. See your doctor as soon as possible.

Day 7

Eat like you live in a Mediterranean country

WHAT IS THE IMPACT ON YOUR HEALTH?

There are numerous countries surrounding the Mediterranean Sea including Greece, Spain, Morocco, southern France and parts of Italy where to varying degrees people follow a traditional diet. It's difficult to be definitive when describing the Mediterranean diet because there are many different customs, foods and cooking methods used throughout the Mediterranean region. But there are some commonalities and, in general, the traditional Mediterranean diet has a strong emphasis on olive oil (not butter), vegetables, nuts, legumes, wholegrains and seafood, and may include moderate amounts of alcohol such as red wine. The end result is a diet low in saturated fat and high in fibre, antioxidants and healthy fats such as omega-3 fatty acids and monounsaturated fats. The health benefits of a Mediterranean diet were first highlighted during research from the mid 1980s which compared the eating habits and wellbeing of people from several different countries. It was found that people who lived in countries bordering the Mediterranean Sea lived healthier and longer lives than those who lived in northern Europe, the United States and Japan. The Greek island of Crete, with its traditional diet rich in unprocessed foods, had the lowest rates of heart disease. In addition to the prevention of heart disease by improving cholesterol and blood pressure, a Mediterranean diet is also associated with a lower risk of arthritis, cancer and age-related memory loss.

SCIENCE SAYS

Fewer bad fats — Mediterranean diets are thought to average around 8 per cent saturated fat, which is 50 per cent less than the average of some industrialised nations. This is because olive oil is used instead of butter and there is a relatively low intake of meat and poultry. Cheese and yoghurts are still consumed in moderation.

Live longer — Research conducted at the University of Athens Medical School found that eating a traditional Mediterranean diet increases longevity. The reduction in mortality was mainly from fewer deaths from both coronary heart disease and cancer.

Fight to maintain tradition — A key aspect of the Mediterranean diet is that it's traditional. According to the

Globocan database, the incidence of diseases like cancer in countries such as Italy increases as the lifestyle and diet of people becomes less traditional. Greater adherence to the traditional Mediterranean diet is associated with a significant reduction in deaths in people with heart disease. However, busy Italians struggling to find the time to prepare a traditional meal can now choose from a growing array of fast-food outlets popping up in cities everywhere.

Mediterranean diet may modify your mid-section — Spanish research published in the journal *Nutrition* found that the more closely subjects followed a Mediterranean dietary pattern, the lower their body fat levels became.

How to eat when you have heart disease — According to research reported in the *Archives of Internal Medicine*, people with heart disease who stick to a Mediterranean-style diet (rich in fish and vegetables and low in saturated fats) were 30 per cent less likely to die during a four-year follow-up compared to those who follow different diets.

Diet can still make a difference, even with medication
A study reported in the *Journal of the American Medical Association* found that a combination of a Mediterranean-style diet and cholesterol-lowering drugs was more effective at lowering cholesterol than either approach alone. Researchers also reported that the Mediterranean diet provided a protective effect against some known side effects from some cholesterol-lowering drugs such as a reduction of antioxidant levels and impaired insulin

regulation. The study was conducted on people who were already taking drugs to keep cholesterol under control.

Just three months makes an impact — A study reported in the *American Journal of Clinical Nutrition* found that eating a Mediterranean-style diet for three months can reduce the risk of heart disease by 15 per cent. Study participants took in fewer kilojoules and consumed more proteins and carbohydrates and less saturated fat and total fat. The subjects also achieved a small but significant drop in body mass index (BMI).

Boost for brain function — According to the *American Journal of Clinical Nutrition*, older adults who stick closely to a traditional Mediterranean diet experience slower rates of cognitive decline as they age. The study was conducted on nearly 4000 adults and the benefits seen were thought to result from reduced markers of oxidative stress.

PRACTICAL TIPS ON HOW TO EAT LIKE YOU LIVE IN A MEDITERRANEAN COUNTRY

It's important to note that the low incidence of heart disease and high life-expectancy rates attributed to the Mediterranean diet are because people ate traditional foods: a good proportion of nutritionally dense plant foods and very little in the way of processed foods. The Mediterranean-style diet is not dependent on one single ingredient and should be seen as a total entity, rather than the sum of its parts. However, each of these parts deserves special mention and I'll explore these individual ingredients in the following sections, including lots of practical tips on how you can enjoy them in your diet. Following are some brief points on the key ingredients of the traditional Mediterranean diet.

- Olive oil — Get to know the different types of olive oil and what they mean for your heart. It's also important to consume olive oil the Mediterranean way: unheated.
- Vegetables — Some Mediterranean countries are known for their open-air markets piled high with locally grown, sun-ripened produce. Vegetables are packed with fibre, nutrients and antioxidants while being low in fat and kilojoules.
- Legumes — Some say the benefits of the Mediterranean diet come from the fact that it is a poor person's diet. Legumes are sometimes described as the poor person's meat. Legumes tend to be overlooked, yet they are rich in fibre and protein, making them the ideal weight-loss and heart-health food. There are plenty of varieties to choose from and they are ideal for soups, salads and dips.
- Nuts and seeds — Once thought of as a dietary 'bad guy', nuts are packed with fibre, protein and healthy fats. There are all kinds of varieties that can be used in many ways, including salads, spreads and as a snack.
- Wholegrains — Breads, pasta and a wide variety of other grains such as polenta, bulgur, couscous and even rice can all be heart-healthy foods depending on how they are processed and the foods you have with them.

- **Seafood** — Fish and other seafood are rich in omega-3 fatty acids, an important and essential fat for heart health. However, eating battered fish or prawns smothered in a creamy dressing will negate any benefits.
- **Alcohol** — Small amounts of alcohol such as red wine can contribute to heart health but a number of conditions apply, such as drinking in moderation and aiming for at least one alcohol-free day per week.

Day 8

Consume more virgin olive oil (unheated)

WHAT IS THE IMPACT ON YOUR HEALTH?

Olive oil is a good source of vitamin E and contains a wide variety of antioxidants depending on the variety. It is also high in monounsaturated fats, which are healthy for your heart. Monounsaturated fats lower your LDL or 'bad' cholesterol levels without lowering your HDL or 'good' cholesterol; potentially, they can raise it. In the fight against atherosclerosis it's important to win the battle between clot-promoting and clot-dissolving factors in your blood vessels. Reducing the amount of bad fats in your diet and replacing them with good fats such as olive oil can help to prevent clot formation and fat being deposited in your arteries. Additional heart health benefits include the reduction of blood pressure. The high levels of antioxidants and flavonoids also help your body fight ageing and disease. As with the relationship between wine and grapes, the flavour of olive oil can vary dramatically depending on the type of olive, the climate, soil and the blend. There are also different processing techniques used to extract the oil from olives, which can alter the impact that it has on your health. The three main types of olive oil are:

- **Extra virgin olive oil/cold pressed olive oil** — This is made from the first pressing after harvest, without the use of excessive heat or chemicals, and the minimal processing involved preserves the flavour, aroma and health benefits. It has more antioxidants (particularly phenols and vitamin E) than other types of olive oil and is remarkably low in acid, giving it the fruitiest, most pronounced flavour.

- **Olive oil/pure olive oil** — After the first pressing more oil is extracted using some heating and processing. It's a middle of the range, all-purpose oil that can be used in salad dressings, sautéing, stir-frying and deep frying. It may also be a combination of refined oil blended with extra virgin oil to replace some of the lost flavour. Refining removes antioxidants so it is not as healthy as extra virgin oil.

- **Light olive oil/extra light olive oil** — This is a highly refined oil resulting from a combination of pressure, heat, filtering and chemical solvents. This process removes most of the colour, odour and taste (hence the name 'light'), making it suitable for frying and baking. This oil is not lower in kilojoules or fat.

Improved hormone balance — Olive oil is known to slow down the absorption of carbohydrates, reducing the body's need to release the fat-storing hormone insulin.

Reduced blood clotting — Research cited in the *American Journal of Clinical Nutrition* has shown that eating foods prepared with virgin olive oil may help ward off harmful blood clots. Olive oil contains phenols that have been shown to fight clotting, and may provide residual protection against the clotting effects of an occasional meal high in saturated fats.

Antioxidants help your heart too — It's thought the unique heart health benefits from olive oil are not due solely to its high content of monounsaturated fatty acids. The high level of antioxidants found in extra virgin oils are also thought to provide a protective effect by preventing LDL cholesterol from oxidising, which is when it damages arteries.

Just a spoonful offers benefits within one week — A study reported in the *European Journal of Clinical Nutrition* found subjects who added just a spoonful or two of extra virgin olive oil (25 millilitres) daily for one week showed less oxidation of LDL (bad) cholesterol and higher levels of antioxidant compounds, particularly phenols, in the blood. According to the researchers, in addition to the LDL-lowering effect of virgin olive oil, an intake of 25 millilitres per day could increase the resistance of LDL to oxidation because it becomes richer in oleic acid and antioxidants.

These benefits could be achieved by including extra virgin olive oil in our daily diet. Those women who consumed at least 30 millilitres of olive oil per day reduced their risk of heart disease by 44 per cent compared to women who only had 15 millilitres or less daily.

Potential cancer-fighting benefits — According to the *Journal of the Federation of American Societies for Experimental Biology,* people who consume plenty of olive oil may be helping to prevent damage to their body cells that can eventually lead to cancer. The researchers believe that the powerful antioxidants in olive oil may be part of the reason that certain cancers, including breast, colon, ovarian and prostate cancers, are less common in Mediterranean countries.

PRACTICAL TIPS ON HOW TO HAVE MORE VIRGIN OLIVE OIL (UNHEATED)

Extra virgin olive oil provides the most benefits to your heart health and longevity, so it is the primary focus of the following tips.

- Extra virgin olive oil is literally the juice of the olive. To maximise the health benefits store it in a cool, dark place for up to 12 months. It should also be tightly capped to minimise exposure to oxygen, which promotes rancidity.
- Extra virgin olive oil is not ideal as a cooking oil because it has a low smoke or heat point. Heating extra virgin olive oil also removes nutrients. Mediterranean people consume their oil at room temperature.

- If you must cook with oil, extra virgin olive oil can tolerate heat to 120°C–190°C (depending on the variety) before the volatile ingredients begin to burn off. Use pure olive oil/olive oil for frying, which is more suited to cooking at higher temperatures.

- Avoid purchasing oil that has been stored or displayed in direct sunlight or in a warm environment. Light and heat are the number one enemies of oil.

- The freshest and youngest oils retain the most health-giving nutrients. The closer to its production you use olive oil, the better. Because olive oil deteriorates with storage, transport and the amount of time after harvest, it may be best to use locally grown olive oil.

- It may be wise to check the national standard for extra virgin olive oil sold in your country. For example, Australian oil labelled 'extra virgin' must meet certain standards, while some imported oils fall short of those standards according to testing conducted by consumer groups.

- Dip bread in extra virgin olive oil instead of using butter or margarine. Butter is high in saturated fats, which have been shown to raise blood cholesterol levels.

- Pour a little extra virgin olive oil over your vegetables after they have been cooked, especially if they have been steamed or microwaved. It's a great way to add flavour to your vegetables without overheating the oil.

- Extra virgin olive oil is the perfect dressing for salads. Try mixing it in equal parts with a little lemon juice or flavoured vinegar, or even on its own to add flavour to your favourite salad.

- Once pasta has been cooked and drained, add a little olive oil to prevent it from clumping and to add extra flavour. This is preferable to adding oil during cooking.
- Add different flavours to olive oil by introducing herbs or spices such as chillies, rosemary or basil. Other flavours that work well include lemon and garlic. The flavours should take around a week to infuse into the oil.
- All fats, including healthy ones like extra virgin olive oil, are high in kilojoules. While extra virgin remains a good choice among fats, don't have more of it just because it's healthy. Olive oil can still contribute to excess body fat if your kilojoule intake exceeds your kilojoule expenditure. Adjust your intake according to your weight-loss goals and activity levels.

Day 9

Include an abundance of fibrous vegetables in your diet

WHAT IS THE IMPACT ON YOUR HEALTH?

There's little doubt that one of the best ways to boost your heart health is to include plenty of fresh vegetables in your diet. Vegetables are packed with fibre, vitamins, minerals and other health-giving nutrients such as antioxidants and phytochemicals. Potassium and folate are just two nutrients that are concentrated in vegetables that have been shown to lower heart disease risk. Fibre helps to slow down and control blood sugar levels while the low kilojoule content of vegetables makes them ideal for weight control. Eating lots of vegetables means there's less room in your stomach for junk foods. All varieties of vegetables are healthy, although some have a lower GI than others. There are two main types of vegetables.

Fibrous (also known as water-rich) vegetables have a high water and low starch content and are generally the best choice for your heart. They are significantly lower in kilojoules than starchy vegetables and have minimal impact on blood sugars because they have a lower GI. Examples of fibrous vegetables include capsicum, zucchini, mushrooms and asparagus.

Starchy vegetables are significantly higher in kilojoules than fibrous vegetables and should be eaten in moderation. They still provide plenty of fibre and nutrients so don't eliminate them from your diet. Examples of starchy vegetables include potatoes, peas, corn and pumpkin.

SCIENCE SAYS

At least one serve a day — A study conducted on over 30,000 women reported in the *American Journal of Clinical Nutrition* found that women who ate at least one daily serving (about 60 grams) of leafy vegetables such as raw lettuce or cooked spinach had a 46 per cent lower chance of developing heart disease than those women who only ate one or two serves per week.

Vegetables lower blood pressure — A six-month study reported in the medical journal *The Lancet* found that adults who consumed at least five servings of fruit and vegetables daily had a 17 per cent reduction in the rate of high blood pressure compared to adults who consumed fewer servings. According to the researchers, a vegetable-rich diet boosts levels of disease-fighting antioxidants in the blood and reduces blood pressure. They added that a higher intake of potassium, which is abundant in many vegetables, is also associated with lower blood pressure.

Vegetables clear your arteries — Research published in the *Journal of Nutrition* has shown that vegetables can help prevent the progression of atherosclerosis in 16 weeks. Mice that were fed a diet full of broccoli, carrots, green beans, corn and peas had 38 per cent less atherosclerosis compared to a group of mice on a vegetable-free diet. The vegetable-eating mice also had lower cholesterol and much lower levels of a protein marker for inflammation.

A high vegetable diet is as good as drugs to lower cholesterol — A study reported in the *Journal of the American Medical Association* found that a diet high in plant foods may be just as good as certain drugs at lowering high cholesterol levels. Subjects with existing high cholesterol levels were put on a high plant and vegetable diet for four weeks. The result was a drop in levels of LDL (bad) cholesterol on par with other subjects taking a class of cholesterol-lowering medication known as statins.

Results in just two weeks — A study labelled the DASH study (Dietary Approaches to Stopping Hypertension) compared subjects on a typical diet with subjects on a low-fat, high fruit and vegetables diet (9 to 10 servings a day). In just two weeks the vegetable eaters saw an impressive drop in blood pressure, reducing their systolic pressure (the higher number) by 11.5 points and the diastolic pressure by 5.5 points.

PRACTICAL TIPS ON EATING MORE VEGETABLES

- Aim for five (for women) to six (for men) servings a day of fibrous vegetables and limit your starchy vegetables to one serving. As a guide to your vegetable intake, one serving is equal to 80 grams or about half a cup of cooked vegetables.

- Examples of fibrous vegetables include asparagus, broccoli, cabbage, cauliflower, zucchini, capsicum, mushrooms, onions, tomato, green beans, alfalfa, bamboo shoots, spinach, leeks, chilli, squash, celery, eggplant, Brussels sprouts, bok choy, snow peas, spring onions, shallots, artichokes, fennel, lettuce, carrots, baby corn and cucumber.

- It's important to note that there's less need to limit starchy vegetables if your weight is under control. Some examples of starchy vegetables include potato, corn pumpkin, peas and sweet potato.

- Vary the methods you use to cook vegetables, for example serving them raw, steamed, microwaved, sautéed, stir-fried, barbecued, grilled or baked. Also be aware that reduced cooking times increases the nutrient and antioxidant content of vegetables.

- Vegetables are often grouped with fruits (that is, 'eat five to seven servings of fruits and vegetables every day'); however, it is important to look at these foods separately. Vegetables, especially the fibrous variety, are much more heart friendly.

- Be aware that minimal cooking time (and minimal exposure to water) helps to maximise the nutrient and antioxidant content of your vegetables.

- Try new types of vegetables regularly because a range of colours and textures makes your diet more interesting and enjoyable. It also increases your exposure to different nutrients.

- Boost your vegetable intake with your next hot breakfast by including foods such as grilled tomatoes and mushrooms, steamed baby spinach and roasted asparagus. Use these instead of bacon, hash browns, breakfast sausages and Hollandaise sauce.

- Include vegetables at lunch in salads and remember that vegetables such as lettuce, cucumber and tomato are a good addition to any salad sandwich. Don't be afraid to add other vegetables on your sandwiches such as sprouts, roasted red capsicum or grated carrot.

- Having two to three healthy vegetarian dinners each week is a sure-fire way to boost your vegetable intake, and also helps to reduce your kilojoule intake at night (which may be beneficial for weight control).

- Have raw vegetables with hummus or salsa as a snack option or alternatively make a dip out of blended vegetables such as roast pumpkin and shallots, sweet potato and cashews or roast capsicum and white beans.

- Frozen vegetables retain a very high percentage of their nutrient content and save time on food preparation. When you consider that fresh vegetables sit at the supermarket, and may remain in your fridge for a while, sometimes frozen vegetables are even richer in nutrients by comparison.

- Canned vegetables can also be convenient but it's advisable to rinse canned vegetables to remove any added salt.
- Don't smother vegetables with butter, sour cream, cheese or salt. Season vegetables with lemon juice or sprinkle with herbs such as oregano, basil, dill or paprika. A little olive oil is also suitable.

Day 10

Eat more beans, peas and lentils

WHAT IS THE IMPACT ON YOUR HEALTH?

A category of food that is often underestimated for its health-giving benefits is legumes (sometimes called pulses). Examples are dried beans, chickpeas and lentils. Lentils come from plants that produce edible pods and are low in saturated fats, even though they are often referred to as the 'poor man's meat'. They are an excellent source of protein, fibre, low GI carbohydrates and essential nutrients. Because of their unique combination of being high in both protein and fibre, lentils are one of the best foods at regulating your blood sugar and insulin levels, and making you feel full. Legumes are rich in soluble fibre, which has been shown to help lower total cholesterol and LDL (bad) cholesterol levels and improve insulin resistance. Legumes contain low levels of sodium and high levels of potassium, calcium and magnesium, a combination that is associated with a reduced risk of heart disease. They are also high in a unique type of fibre called resistant starch, which is great for weight control (see Day 28 for more information). Increasing your legume consumption is an important dietary change you can make to reduce the risk of heart disease.

SCIENCE SAYS

Loaded with antioxidants — Research published in the *Journal of Agriculture and Food Chemistry* found that black beans are as rich in antioxidants as cranberries and 10 times higher in antioxidants than oranges. Among different types of bean, the researchers found that the darker a bean's seed coat, the higher its level of antioxidant activity. Black beans were the richest in antioxidant activity, followed in descending order by red, brown, yellow and white beans.

Beans means heart health — A study reported in the *Archives of Internal Medicine* found that people who consumed high quantities of legumes had, on average, lower systolic blood pressure and lower total cholesterol and body mass index than those who consumed fewer legumes. What's more, those who consumed legumes at least four times a week had a 22 per cent reduced risk of heart disease compared to those who ate legumes less than once a week.

Folate in legumes is a heart helper — Legumes are a rich source of folate, a nutrient which helps to break down homocysteine (a known risk factor for heart disease). For example, one cup of cooked black beans provides around two-thirds of your daily folate needs.

Legumes help you get leaner — Researchers reported in the *Journal of Nutrition and Metabolism* that replacing just 5.4 per cent of carbohydrates with resistant starch (for instance by eating more legumes) increased fat burning by 23 per cent. In other words, legumes change the way your body uses fuel. You may not necessarily burn too many extra kilojoules but you will use a higher proportion of fat as fuel compared to glucose. Resistant starch in a meal is associated with less fat storage after that meal and, over the long term, this could help to reduce stored body fat.

Legumes reduce the need for insulin — Consuming pulses may lessen the amount of insulin required to control blood sugar levels. The slow rise in blood sugar after eating legumes (they are a very low GI food) can help to prevent the release of the fat-storing hormone insulin.

PRACTICAL TIPS ON EATING MORE BEANS, PEAS AND LENTILS

Beans, peas and lentils are conveniently available in cans or in packets for soaking and are a great partner for many meals and cuisines. Following are some ideas on how you could include more beans, peas and lentils in your diet.

- Look for ways to include legumes in your diet at least four to five times a week. One serving is roughly three heaped tablespoons of beans.
- Canned varieties of pulses such as chickpeas and beans save the hassle of soaking and are just as beneficial. Lentils, black-eyed peas and split peas don't need to be soaked at all and are terrific in soups.
- Hummus is a very versatile food. In a food processor combine a tin of drained chickpeas with lemon juice, cumin, garlic salt, fresh herbs and low-fat natural yoghurt for a tasty spread. You can also follow the same method, using cannellini beans instead of chickpeas, for a tasty white bean dip. Sprinkle with paprika for some added spice.
- Replace some of the meat in your recipes with beans, peas or lentils.
- Lentils are relatively quick and easy to prepare and are good at absorbing a variety of flavours from other foods and seasonings. Use red lentils in soups, pasta sauces, burgers, stews and curries or make your own dhal. Add them pureed or whole.
- Use red kidney beans in shepherd's pie or chilli con carne.
- Use black-eyed peas and split peas in soups.
- Use pinto or refried beans in burritos.
- Add white cannellini beans or chickpeas to a minted salad.
- Have a warm breakfast including baked beans.
- Add beans and chickpeas to salads.
- If you are concerned that beans, peas and lentils give you gas, try adding mustard seeds to them during cooking. This is thought to reduce the gas-producing effect of pulses.

Day 11

Include some nuts and seeds in your diet

WHAT IS THE IMPACT ON YOUR HEALTH?

Nuts and seeds are packed with protein, fibre and a number of nutrients that could be responsible for protection against heart disease including vitamin E, antioxidants, magnesium and arginine. They are low in saturated fats and rich in polyunsaturated and monounsaturated fats, the types of fats that actually reduce cardiovascular disease risk. Nuts and seeds also contain naturally occurring cholesterol-lowering compounds called plant sterols. Many of the heart health benefits attributed to nuts stem from the fact that they help lower your cholesterol and these benefits extend to men and women of all ages and races. Nuts are also a good hunger-buster, and may even prevent weight gain. As they are high in protein, unsaturated fats and fibre they can help you to feel full and therefore possibly reduce your intake of other high-kilojoule foods afterwards. This is because nuts have a low GI, helping to slow digestion and stabilise blood glucose levels. In addition, the high nutrient content of nuts may stimulate fat metabolism, improving your body's ability to burn kilojoules. There is also a theory that people don't chew nuts well, so the body may fail to absorb a portion of the kilojoule content. The flip side of the coin is that nuts and seeds are very high in fat and kilojoules and may contribute to weight gain depending on the serving size consumed.

SCIENCE SAYS

Go nuts four times a week — A study conducted on 31,000 people reported in the *Archives of Internal Medicine* found that people who ate nuts more than four times a week were 40 per cent less likely to die of coronary heart disease than those who ate nuts less than once a week.

Go nutty even more — A study reported in the *British Medical Journal* found that frequent nut consumption protects your heart. Subjects who ate nuts five or more times a week (equivalent to around 30 grams, or two tablespoons worth each time) had a 50 per cent reduction in the risk of coronary disease compared to those who ate them twice a week or less.

Even twice a week has benefits — A study reported in the *Archives of Internal Medicine* on men who ate nuts at least twice a week found that they had half the rate of sudden cardiac death as men who rarely or never ate nuts.

Cholesterol lowering — A study published in the *Journal of American College of Nutrition* showed that nuts have a beneficial effect on blood cholesterol levels. When 100 grams of almonds a day were added to the diets of both men and women with elevated cholesterol levels, their cholesterol was lowered by between 7 and 10 per cent in nine weeks.

All nuts are beneficial — According to the journal *Clinical Cardiology*, almonds and walnuts may be most effective at lowering cholesterol; macadamia nuts may be the least beneficial. However, all nut varieties have been shown to contribute to lowering cholesterol levels, namely LDL cholesterol, by between 10 and 15 per cent.

Walnuts ranked high in antioxidants — In a report presented to the 241st national meeting of the American Chemical Society, walnuts were found to contain more antioxidants than other popular nuts — and these antioxidants were considered more potent. A handful of walnuts contains almost twice the amount of antioxidants as an equivalent quantity of other nuts such as almonds, peanuts, pistachios, hazelnuts, Brazil nuts, cashews, macadamias and pecans.

Nuts reduce triglycerides — An eight-week study published in the *Journal of the American College of Nutrition* found that reducing participants' dietary fat intake by 500 calories and replacing them with 500 calories of peanuts lowered their triglyceride levels by 24 per cent. Triglycerides are a marker of fat in the blood and are a known risk factor for cardiovascular disease.

Nuts combine well with a Mediterranean diet — A study published in the *Archives of Internal Medicine* shows that the Mediterranean diet, with the addition of nuts, may help manage a range of heart disease symptoms. The study found that adding nuts was even more effective than adding olive oil in reducing waist circumference, triglycerides and blood pressure levels in older adults who were at a high risk of heart disease.

Flaxseeds cut cholesterol — According to the *Journal of Clinical Endocrinology and Metabolism*, flaxseeds may help to reduce levels of cholesterol by 6 per cent in post-menopausal women. Volunteers in this study consumed 40 grams of ground flaxseeds daily for three months.

PRACTICAL TIPS ON HOW TO INCLUDE SOME NUTS AND SEEDS IN YOUR DIET

- Stick to raw and roasted nuts (not in oil) that have been minimally processed. Roasting nuts in oil, sprinkling them with salt or covering them with chocolate or sugar can negate any of the health benefits associated with nuts.
- When you eat nuts and seeds, watch your portion size because they are easy to overeat. Aim for a small handful (approximately a quarter of a cup) four to five times per week. Place each serving of nuts in a small zip-lock bag for portion control and easy transport.

- Try to choose from a wide variety of nuts when you are looking to include small amounts of nuts in your diet. These include cashews, pecans, walnuts, pine nuts, pistachios, macadamias, hazelnuts, Brazil nuts, almonds, chestnuts and peanuts (although technically peanuts are a legume).
- Some of the seeds you can add to your diet include pumpkin, sesame, linseed, sunflower and poppy.
- LSA (which stands for linseeds, sunflower kernels and almonds) is a ground-up mix of all three ingredients. It is a good source of protein and omega-3 fats that you can sprinkle over breakfast cereal, muesli and low-fat natural yoghurt or in smoothies. It is best stored in the fridge.
- Ground nuts can be stirred into a number of recipes such as dukkah, pancakes or muffins or mixed with herbs and used as a coating for baked chicken or fish.
- Nuts and seeds are delicious in stir-fries, soups, salads, smoothies, casseroles, breakfast cereal and yoghurt.
- The best way to add nuts and seeds to your diet is to eat them instead of other foods that are high in saturated fat. For example, sprinkle some pine nuts over your cooked vegetables instead of adding a dob of butter.
- Start your evening meal with a few nuts. Eating nuts or seeds before dinner or in an early course, such as in a soup or starter salad, produces a feeling of fullness that may reduce your kilojoule intake later.
- To maximise the nutrient value of nuts it may be best to store them in an airtight container in the refrigerator. This is because the delicate oils in nuts can become rancid easily

(producing free radicals). For this reason it may also be best to purchase nuts in small quantities to guarantee freshness. In addition, chopped nuts deteriorate much quicker than whole nuts.

- If you are concerned about your calcium intake be aware that almonds provide the most calcium of any non-animal food. Almonds are available commercially whole, sliced, slivered or as a nut meal to use in baking, and even as a milk.

- A little peanut butter now and again is OK but watch the sugar and salt content and have it on bread by itself instead of adding butter or margarine.

Day 12

Eat more wholegrains

WHAT IS THE IMPACT ON YOUR HEALTH?

The processing of grains has led to the development of a wide variety of foods such as pasta, bread, breakfast cereals, baked goods and white rice, to name a few. But manipulating the components of the grain that we eat can have a drastic impact on our health. Processing removes the outer layer of the grain (the bran) and may also remove the seed or germ. What's left is the kilojoule-dense centre that flour is made from. Much of the fibre is gone (this is the part that fills you up and slows down absorption), along with the nutrients needed to help digest the grain and nourish your body. By contrast, wholegrains are consumed in their natural state, and are richer in fibre, protein, B vitamins, minerals and antioxidants. They contain all the original parts of the entire grain seed, unchanged from when they were growing in a field. Foods made from wholegrains that have been processed (cracked, crushed, rolled, lightly pearled or cooked) can still be considered wholegrain if they contain the same rich balance of nutrients found in the original wholegrain seed. Some common types of grain that can be eaten whole or that are used to make wholegrain foods include wheat, barley, brown rice, buckwheat, bulgur, corn, oats and rye. Due to their high fibre and nutrient content, eating wholegrains is associated with a lower risk of heart disease, high blood pressure, bowel cancer and type 2 diabetes. Wholegrains take longer to digest, filling you up more and providing longer lasting energy. They also help to prevent a spike in blood sugar, reducing the need for insulin and, ultimately, reducing the storage of body fat.

SCIENCE SAYS

Three portions lowers blood pressure — According to the *American Journal of Clinical Nutrition*, the daily consumption of three portions of wholegrain foods is linked to lower cardiovascular disease risk by lowering blood pressure. The study found that systolic blood pressure (the high number) was significantly reduced, while cholesterol concentrations decreased slightly.

Heart help from wholegrains — According to the *Journal of the American Medical Association*, people over 65 were less likely to develop cardiovascular disease if they ate fibre-rich cereals or dark breads such as wheat, rye or pumpernickel. The researchers speculated that people with the lowest fibre intake could boost their heart health by eating just two extra slices of wholegrain bread each day.

Oats help with weight loss — A recent study conducted by the Rippe Lifestyle Institute in the United States looked at the weight-loss effect of eating oats for breakfast as part of an overall reduced-kilojoule weight-loss plan. It was found the subjects lost significant amounts of weight and body fat when compared to control subjects who didn't eat oats. Over the 12 weeks of the study, the oat-eating subjects (who also walked for 15 to 30 minutes a day) reduced their waist circumference by 5 centimetres and reduced their body fat, level by 5 per cent. It was also highlighted that 80 per cent of the weight loss was from loss of fat with lean muscle mass largely preserved.

Oats reduce the need for medication — A study reported in *The Journal of Family Practice* found that the daily consumption of wholegrain oat cereal reduces blood pressure, and in patients already taking blood pressure medication allows a decrease in dosage. Subjects with existing high blood pressure were given 137 grams of oat cereal daily, which contains 12 grams of total fibre and 6 grams of soluble fibre. Over the course of the 12-week study, LDL (bad) cholesterol dropped by 16 per cent, blood glucose levels improved significantly and 73 per cent of subjects were able to reduce their blood pressure medication. These results were far more impressive than those of a group who consumed 137 grams of wheat cereal daily (approximately 3 grams of total fibre and 1 gram of soluble fibre). Of the wheat group, only 42 per cent were able to decrease their dose of blood pressure medication and there was no significant change in LDL cholesterol levels.

Oats as a cholesterol-lowering superfood — According to researchers at the University of Kentucky College of Medicine, the consumption of oats can help lower LDL (bad) cholesterol without adverse effects on HDL (good) cholesterol. It's also thought oats may contain unique compounds that can help reduce early hardening of the arteries.

Do as the doctors do — Research known as the Physicians' Health Study, which collected data from over 10,500 doctors, found that those who ate wholegrain cereal every day (defined as a minimum of 25 per cent bran or oat content) were 28 per cent less likely to develop heart failure compared to non-wholegrain breakfast eaters.

Wholegrains are a cluster buster — A study reported in the *American Journal of Clinical Nutrition* found that older adults (aged between 60 and 98) who regularly eat wholegrains like high-fibre cereals and cooked oats may be less likely to develop metabolic syndrome, a cluster of conditions that raise the risk of heart attack and stroke. These conditions include high blood pressure, high cholesterol, high blood sugar levels and abdominal obesity.

PRACTICAL TIPS ON HOW TO EAT MORE WHOLEGRAINS

- Aim for two to four servings of wholegrain foods each day, including bread, rolls and flatbreads, breakfast cereal, wholemeal pasta, brown rice and couscous.
- Experiment with the lesser-known types of wholegrain foods such as quinoa, millet, sorghum, spelt, wild rice and amaranth.
- While whole grains are a better choice than processed grains they still contain more kilojoules and less nutrients per gram than vegetables. Try not to eat grain-based foods at the expense of vegetables.
- While wholegrain foods offer unique heart health benefits, it is still important to manage your portion sizes.
- Make sure your bread has the least amount of processing. Ideally, choose whole grains, rye and pumpernickel over white bread. Wholemeal and high-fibre white breads lie in between. It's also important to choose wisely the toppings you use. Be sure to minimise or eliminate butter (high in saturated fat) and margarine (chemically altered fats).
- Look for a breakfast cereal that contains whole grains such as oats, whole wheat or barley. When looking at packaged cereals check the nutrition information panel on your breakfast cereal box to compare the fibre content. Those that contain bran and whole grains will generally have the highest fibre content.
- Try to minimise your intake of highly processed, man-made grain products like white bread, white rice, white flour and low-fibre breakfast cereals.

- While wholemeal pasta is a healthier choice than white pasta, most types of pasta have a low GI due to the type of starch used.
- Enjoy whole grains in salads, like cracked wheat in tabbouleh. You can also add whole grains such as pearl barley to soup.
- If you are a little unsure as to how to prepare whole grains, search the internet for wholegrain recipes and ideas.

Day 13

Eat more fish and seafood

HOW CAN IT BENEFIT YOUR HEALTH?

Healthy fats in your diet provide a wide range of nutrients. The human body can manufacture some of the important fats it needs, while others can only be obtained from your diet. The type of fat in seafood (known as omega-3 fatty acid) is one such 'essential' dietary fat and it has a wide range of health benefits. The protective effects to your heart include:

- reduced blood clotting and improved blood flow
- reduced blood triglyceride levels
- reduced risk of developing an irregular heart rhythm
- reduced arterial hardness
- reduced blood pressure.

The additional benefits include reduced inflammation, mood elevation, reduced food cravings and improved energy levels, which all have secondary benefits for your heart. Another role that fish and seafood play in boosting your health is by improving what's called omega balancing. The human body is thought to function best with a 2:1 ratio of omega-6 to omega-3 fats. However, western diets typically have ratios of 10 or even 20 to 1. It's thought that excessive levels of omega-6 fatty acids from a high intake of vegetable oils and processed foods may increase the risk of a number of diseases and depression. If your intake of omega-6 fats is too high it can compete with the omega-3 fats and stop them providing their wide range of benefits.

SCIENCE SAYS

Eat fish at least twice a week — The Nurses' Health Study conducted on over 5000 women found that those who reported eating fish between two and four times per week had their risk of heart disease reduced by 36 per cent compared to women who ate fish less frequently. This study was reported in the journal *Circulation*.

Daily fish lowers blood pressure — A study reported in the *American Journal of Clinical Nutrition* showed that a kilojoule-restricted diet combined with daily fish consumption was highly effective in reducing blood pressure, lowering triglyceride levels while increasing 'good' cholesterol levels and in improving glucose tolerance.

Benefits from dark flesh seafood — A study at Tufts University showed that eating at least two servings of fish each week was linked to slower worsening of heart lesions. The findings were particularly true for tuna and dark meat fish such as salmon, sardines and mackerel.

Omega-3 fats protect the heart — A study published in *The New England Journal of Medicine* found men with no existing heart disease were 81 per cent less likely to experience sudden death when their blood levels of omega-3 fatty acids were high regardless of their age, smoking habits or the amount of other types of fatty acids in their blood.

Cut heart attack risk in half — A study published in the *Journal of the American Medical Association* reported that women who consumed at least five servings of fish a week lowered their risk of heart disease by more than one-third, and also cut their risk of heart attack by half over a 16-year period.

Never too old to benefit — A study conducted at the University of Washington's Cardiovascular Health Research Unit found that the benefits of eating fish like tuna, salmon or sardines don't have an upper age limit. Subjects (who were all over the age of 65) who consumed fatty fish, even just once a week, lowered their risk of a fatal heart attack by 44 per cent compared to those who did not eat fish. The benefits did not extend to fried fish.

Baked, not fried — A study conducted on over 4800 people, and reported in the journal *Circulation*, found that baked or broiled fish (not fried), helped reduce the risk of arterial fibrillation. Subjects who ate fish one to four times per week had a 28 per cent lower risk, compared to those who ate fish less than once a month.

Improvement in just seven weeks — A study published in the *American Journal of Clinical Nutrition* found the omega-3 fatty acids present in fish helped to reduce the risk of heart attack by softening the arteries. There was a significant improvement in arterial elasticity after just seven weeks.

Fish may be less fattening — Eating fish may be of secondary benefit to your heart according to a preliminary research finding that omega-3 fats may be unlikely to be stored as body fat. While this is exciting, this study was conducted on animals so further research is needed.

PRACTICAL TIPS ON EATING MORE FISH AND SEAFOOD

- Fish and seafood are a diverse, healthy and incredibly delicious food category. All seafood contains varying amounts of omega-3 fatty acids, yet oily, cold-water fish such as mackerel, salmon, trout, anchovies, tuna, sardines, herring and gem fish are some of the richest sources.
- Canned fish like sardines, salmon, herrings and tuna are also good sources of omega-3 fatty acids. Canned fish is ideal for sandwiches and wraps.
- Try to include at least two servings of omega-3 rich fish and seafood every week.
- When preparing and cooking seafood look for healthy cooking methods such as baking, grilling or barbecuing. Any

benefit from the consumption of seafood is dramatically reduced if it is battered, fried or swimming in butter or cream.

- Look for recipes that use fish or shellfish in your stir-fries, salads, soups, pasta recipes and casseroles. Barbecue squid and octopus are also ideal in green salads.
- Find creative ways to add flavour to fish and seafood by using herbs, spices and marinades (garlic, lemon juice, soy) instead of using too much fat or salt.
- When cooking steaks on the barbecue, it doesn't always have to be red meat. Why not try a fish steak, using swordfish, tuna or salmon?
- A less potent type of omega-3 fatty acid is found in a variety of plant foods, including tofu, flaxseed, walnuts and green vegetables. But you need to eat a larger amount of plant-based omega-3 fatty acids to get the same benefit as the marine sources offer.
- Fish oil capsules are an alternative for people who don't like eating fish or seafood. It's not completely clear if isolated fish oil supplements reproduce the exact benefits of actually eating fish but it's likely there is some benefit.

Day 14

Drink only moderate amounts of alcohol (and have alcohol-free days)

WHAT IS THE IMPACT ON YOUR HEALTH?

While drinking in moderation can have some health benefits, drinking too much can have the opposite effect. It's a classic case of where a little is good but a lot is not. It's thought moderate amounts of alcohol benefit the heart by thinning the blood, and increase 'good' cholesterol levels. However, it can be difficult to describe what is a safe amount of alcohol to drink because there are many variables to consider. These variables include weight, gender, speed of consumption, the type of alcohol you are drinking, if you are eating while drinking, and your age. For example, in middle-aged and older adults, consuming one or two alcoholic drinks a day is associated with a lower risk of heart disease compared to non-drinkers. For younger adults alcohol provides little benefit and is actually associated with a higher risk of trauma. It's not recommended that anyone start drinking or drink more frequently to boost heart health. It's important to recognise that diet and exercise play a much more significant role in preventing heart disease. But alcohol creates a pleasant, relaxed feeling that many people enjoy and it can be part of a healthy lifestyle if it's consumed in moderation. See the practical tips below for a specific definition of what constitutes drinking in moderation.

Alcohol and your weight

Another way that alcohol impacts upon your heart health is that it can trigger weight gain. Alcohol is high in kilojoules but since they can't be stored, the kilojoules from alcohol have to be used as fuel before your body can burn off any food kilojoules. In other words, alcohol slows down, even prevents, the foods you eat from being burnt off, especially those you consume with alcohol. Other negatives are that alcohol also increases your appetite, reduces your willpower to say no to unhealthy foods and often comes with extra kilojoules from mixers (such as soft drinks, energy drinks or fruit juice). If alcohol is consumed in excess, the resultant hangover the following day may lead to fat bingeing and inactivity, neither of which is good for weight control.

SCIENCE SAYS

Alcohol and abdominal fat — A study published in the *Journal of Nutrition* found that drinking alcohol has a strong influence on the accumulation of abdominal fat, a known risk factor for cardiovascular diseases. The researchers found that, in both men and women, the more drinks consumed per drinking day, the higher the abdominal fat measurement.

Binge drinking and belly fat — A study published in the *Journal of Nutrition* found that it's not only the total amount of alcohol that you drink each week that's important but the way that you drink it. Binge drinkers (defined as individuals who have more than three to four drinks per drinking session) had more abdominal fat than people who consumed the same amount of alcohol in the course of a week but consumed small amounts on a regular basis.

Don't drink and drive — Alcohol is a depressant to the central nervous system, reducing reaction time and impairing judgment, which increases the likelihood and severity of trauma. Injury and trauma are a major cause of hospital visits, with alcohol playing a significant role. Research has shown that 38.6 per cent of all traffic deaths involve alcohol-impaired drivers.

A tick for moderate drinking — A study reported by *The New England Journal of Medicine* found that half an alcoholic drink every second day (wine, whisky or beer) reduced the risk of heart attacks by a third.

Another tick for moderate drinking — Findings reported in the journal *Arteriosclerosis, Thrombosis and Vascular Biology* suggest that people who drink one to six alcoholic beverages per week have the least amount of atherosclerosis, while people who consumed 14 or more drinks per week had the most.

Alcohol and stroke risk — A report in the *Journal of the American Medical Association* found that moderate drinkers who consume one to two alcoholic drinks a day reduce their risk of having a stroke. However, consuming more than five drinks a day has the opposite effect, doubling a person's risk of stroke.

Heart boost from cutting back — The *American Journal of Hypertension* reported that habitual heavy drinkers (defined as individuals who have at least four drinks a day) who cut their alcohol intake in half for just three weeks experienced a drop in both blood pressure and heart rate.

It's not about the drink — The *American Journal of Clinical Nutrition* suggests that the heart health benefits experienced by moderate wine drinkers may have more to do with their heart healthy lifestyles rather than any specific components in the wine itself. For example, wine drinkers tend to be thinner, eat more vegetables, exercise more, drink alcohol with food and smoke less compared to those who prefer beer or spirits.

PRACTICAL TIPS ON HOW TO MANAGE YOUR ALCOHOL INTAKE

The following tips are a guide to drinking in moderation allowing you to take advantage of the heart health benefits of alcohol.

- Moderate drinking is defined as consuming no more than one standard drink a day for women and up to two standard drinks a day for men. A standard drink is defined as 10 grams or 12.7 millilitres of alcohol. This equates roughly to 30 millilitres of straight spirits, one small glass (285 millilitres or a middie) of full strength beer, one large glass (425 millilitres or a schooner) of light beer, or a 100-millilitre glass of wine.

- Wine can be hard to measure and it's not uncommon for people to pour more than a standard glass (100 millilitres) of wine. This is especially true when wine is served in a big glass or when your glass keeps getting topped up. Get to know what makes up a standard serving in the glass you typically drink from.

- Drink slowly. Sculling down your alcoholic drinks is not considered drinking in moderation.

- Aim to include two to four alcohol-free days (and nights) each week.

- Don't binge drink. Binge drinking is defined as consuming more than three drinks a day for women, and more than four drinks a day for men. Don't assume it's healthy to save up your daily totals and consume them all at once. Also, recognise that anything more than moderate drinking can be harmful to your health.

- When you consume alcoholic beverages, try drinking a glass of water between each alcoholic drink. You can also add ice to drinks like wine and alcoholic cider to water them down, especially in the warmer months.

- Have a plan when you drink socially. Space out your drinks, avoid getting in shouts and offer to drive to release any social pressure. You can still enjoy the company of others and they can enjoy yours without binge drinking.

- Most low-carbohydrate drinks are still high in kilojoules. The best choice is the lower alcohol drinks such as light beers, shandies, half spirits and spritzers (wine and soda).

- Drinking alcohol while eating food slows down its absorption. But the foods often associated with alcohol can be high in bad fats and salt, such as pies, hot dogs, sausage rolls, cheese, dips and nibblies. Try to make the foods that you consume with alcohol heart healthy.

- Try to be active on the days you drink alcohol. This can help compensate for the extra kilojoules consumed.

- Don't fall for the trap of thinking that red wine is healthy. While the antioxidants in red wine are beneficial for cardiovascular health, the same benefits can be found from eating fruit and vegetables or drinking grape juice. There are no significant health advantages from choosing to drink red wine over other types of alcohol.

Day 15

Improve your management of stress

WHAT IS THE IMPACT ON YOUR HEALTH?

Stress can have a dramatic influence on your heart health and quality of life. If you are unhappy with your job, your relationship, your children, your finances, your relatives, your neighbours or there are any other worries that dominate your thinking, it's hard to prioritise health. The stress hormones adrenalin and cortisol are released, triggering a raft of changes designed to help your body in a fight or flight situation. Your heart rate and blood pressure are increased as more blood and nutrients are delivered to your muscles. Your blood becomes more sticky and prone to clots as the body prepares for possible injury, while blood fats and sugar are released to provide fuel. These changes are ideal when we are stressed during exercise or in a life-threatening situation. But when you are usually fairly inactive and these stresses occur over the long term, your risk of heart disease increases. Prolonged stress is harmful, builds tension and can lead to burnout and depression, having a negative impact on all aspects of your health. A vicious cycle can arise where stress makes you feel lethargic, leading to inactivity and bad food choices. During times of stress, many people may also find it hard to resist high-fat foods such as chocolate, ice-cream, biscuits, cakes and pastries. While stress can trigger weight loss in some people, others gain it, which can make that individual even more depressed. Learning to manage your stress can help to counter some of these negative effects of stress and prevent the build-up of stress in the first place.

SCIENCE SAYS

More stress equals more weight — A study from Rush University Medical Center found that the more stressors a woman reported, the more weight she had gained over four years, even after taking into account variables that influence weight such as diet, exercise, smoking and age.

Stress leads to temptation — A study reported in the *Journal of Social and Clinical Psychology* found that during times of stress people find it hardest to resist unhealthy temptations. The researchers found that during periods of high stress, the subjects ate less healthy foods, drank more high-caffeine drinks and slept less. Stress appeared to cause a relapse in behaviours that were previously under control. During times of stress, people could only cope with so much and were particularly vulnerable to a loss of self-control.

Stress linked to blood vessel problems — A study published in the journal *Arteriosclerosis, Thrombosis, and Vascular Biology* has shown that anxiety may accelerate the development of atherosclerosis and put people at a higher risk of heart disease and heart attack. The researchers quizzed over 700 people to assess their anxiety levels and performed several scans over time to monitor any fatty deposits on the inner walls of arteries. It was found that men with sustained anxiety showed both a higher rate of development of atherosclerosis and increased blood vessel thickness when compared with men who were not anxious. Women showed an increased blood vessel thickness only.

Stress impedes blood flow — The journal *Circulation* has discovered that stress appears to inhibit the ability of blood vessels to expand, a phenomenon that may help explain why extremely stressful events can precipitate heart attacks. After scanning healthy people as they performed a stressful task, it was found that blood flow was restricted by up to 50 per cent for about 45 minutes. The test also caused both blood pressure and heart rate to temporarily increase.

Depression linked to heart risk — According to the *American Journal of Cardiology,* men suffering from pronounced depression run a higher risk of developing heart disease than men who are less depressed or not depressed. According to the researchers, people who are depressed may have higher levels of stress hormones in their bloodstream, and this may raise their blood pressure. In addition, depressed people are more likely to smoke, to eat unhealthy diets and to be sedentary — all factors that increase heart disease risk.

Stress and inflammation — A study reported in the *American Journal of Cardiology* has shown that depressed individuals have higher levels of inflammatory proteins and other 'markers' in the blood. Negative emotions like depressed mood, anxiety and pessimism were associated with greater heart risks, even when other key factors like abdominal obesity, high blood pressure and insulin resistance were taken into account.

Stress management helps the heart — A study reported in the *American Journal of Cardiology* found that adding stress management to routine heart disease treatment might lessen some patients' long-term risk of complications. The study found that men with heart disease who underwent four months of stress management training had fewer adverse cardiac events and less medical expenditures over a five-year period. The stress management sessions taught people ways to control negative emotions and thoughts, techniques for muscle relaxation and other stress-calming tactics.

PRACTICAL TIPS TO HELP YOU STRESS LESS AND RELAX MORE

It's not possible to completely eliminate stress but you can learn to manage and control it, reducing its harmful effects on your physical and mental health. Spending more time relaxing and improving your relaxation skills is helpful at countering the harmful effects of stress. Stress management involves a range of strategies designed to reduce stress or prevent it from occurring. Here are some suggestions that may help.

- Awareness is vital in addressing stress. People cope with stress differently, so try to identify what causes you stress and how you react to it. Determine what events and specific situations trigger feelings of stress. When are you most vulnerable to stress? Are there repetitive situations that drain you of energy or a combination of situations that accumulate to stress you out? For example, are you disorganised or do you have issues with a colleague at work? Do you become nervous or physically upset when stressed and, if so, in what specific ways? For example, can you identify areas in your body where muscle tension bothers you.

- Try to identify what you can change. Can you change your stressors by avoiding or eliminating them completely? Can you reduce their intensity by extending them over a period of time or shorten your exposure to the stressor? Re-evaluate your goals and develop some pre-planned methods for dealing with stressful situations.

- The degree of control that you feel you have over your life is very important. Improving your time management and organisational skills may help to prevent a stressful crisis and contribute to better sleep.
- Set priorities and allocate your time towards the most valuable, rewarding tasks. There's never enough time to do everything but there is always enough time to do the most important things. When faced with a new email or piece of paper, apply the FAT principle (File, Act or Toss). It helps to prevent clutter or wasted time looking for misplaced information.
- Get better at saying 'no', especially if you are vulnerable to stress. By being better at managing your time and knowing your priorities, it becomes clearer what tasks are important and what are time wasters. Get to know your limits and avoid taking on too much at once. Rather than looking for ways to squeeze more into the day, find ways to leave things out.

Day 16

Include more incidental movement in your day

WHAT IS THE IMPACT ON YOUR HEALTH?

There are two main categories of physical activity that can impact upon your heart health. Day 6 has addressed what's known as planned exercise, which is scheduled, progressive, organised and constant. Another important type of exercise for cardiovascular health is called incidental movement. This is sometimes referred to as spontaneous physical activity or random acts of movement. It involves short bursts of activity that you accumulate over the course of the day such as walking from the car to work, to the bank or around the house. This type of activity doesn't have to involve breaking into a sweat, red-faced puffing or the need to shower immediately afterwards. While it might seem trivial it's the reduction in incidental movement from labour-saving devices that is thought to be one of the leading contributors to the increasing rates of obesity around the developed world. The use of dishwashers, clothes dryers, washing machines, cordless phones, remote controls, escalators, lifts, home delivery, electronic can openers, electronic tooth brushes and drive-in food service, to name a few, is commonplace, both at work and in the home. Including more incidental movement in your day helps to compensate for the inactivity that has been engineered into modern life. While planned movement is a better fat burner (especially as you get fitter), there are still significant benefits to be had from simply moving more in everyday life.

SCIENCE SAYS

Even a short walk helps the heart — Research presented to a conference of the American Heart Association has shown that obese people who are relatively inactive may have trouble dissolving potentially deadly blood clots, but moderate exercise a few times per week appears to help restore that ability. The study found obese, sedentary people are less able than individuals of normal weight to produce and release a clot-busting substance known as tissue plasminogen activator (t-PA), the body's primary defence mechanism against the formation of blood clots. But after exercise, the ability of some obese people to release t-PA became similar to the lean, age-matched counterparts in the study.

10,000 steps is a helpful guide — According to research published in the journal *Sports Medicine*, taking 10,000 steps is the recommended daily step goal for weight control and cardiovascular health. The 10,000 steps goal also puts a focus on the accumulation of activity across the whole day, incorporating both planned and incidental activity.

Accumulating exercise lowers blood pressure — A study reported in the *American Journal of Clinical Nutrition* has shown that short bouts of exercise can be just as effective for heart health as longer, continuous bouts. The study found that a group who performed multiple short (3 minutes) bouts of brisk walking (30 minutes in total) throughout a day experienced the same benefits of lowered tricylglycerol levels (blood fats) and systolic blood pressure as a group that performed one continuous 30-minute brisk walk.

Accumulating exercise lowers cholesterol — A study that appeared in the *International Journal of Obesity* compared a group who performed continuous walking (30 minutes three times a week) with a group who performed intermittent exercise (15 minutes, twice a day on five days a week). HDL (good) cholesterol increased significantly for both groups — by 15 per cent for the continuous group and 9 per cent for the intermittent group. In other measures, both groups saw a significant reduction in the need for insulin and a boost in aerobic fitness. Both groups also lost weight, although the continuous group lost more. This study was performed on previously sedentary, moderately overweight subjects.

Mild exercise cuts heart-related deaths — According to the guidelines for physical activity in people with heart disease published in *The Medical Journal of Australia*, gentle exercise performed daily could cut death rates by a third, and improve the lives of millions of people living with cardiovascular disease. According to the researchers behind the guidelines, 30 minutes of mild exercise a day would also lower blood pressure and decrease the need for medication. Other benefits could include fewer hospitalisations, less spending on health care, improved state of wellbeing and a reduction in anxiety and depression.

PRACTICAL TIPS TO INCLUDING MORE INCIDENTAL MOVEMENT IN YOUR DAY

- In most cases the type of activity you will undertake to accumulate extra movement in your day will be walking. Walking is ideal as it is accessible, free and requires no equipment or coordination, and can be incorporated into daily life with little risk of injury.
- Performing short bouts of exercise can be as effective for heart health and even weight control as long sessions, especially if you are unfit or overweight. Including a few short bouts of walking into your day is also a good strategy if you are time poor.
- Whatever your mode of transport to school, work or study, aim to include some walking as part of your journey. For

example, if you catch public transport, get off several stops before your destination. If suitable footwear is a concern, a small backpack will allow you to carry a change of shoes, and a water bottle if needed.

- Whenever you get the opportunity take the stairs instead of the escalator or lift.
- When parking your car, pick a distant spot in the parking lot so you have to walk further than usual. You'll also probably find it easier to get a parking space.
- Don't drive a car when you can ride a bike and don't ride a bike when you can walk.
- If you have a busy work schedule that makes it hard to exercise, use your lunch break to go for a short walk.
- Do laborious tasks for yourself when you can, such as cleaning, gardening and washing your car. You'll save money and burn off extra kilojoules.
- Do your housework more vigorously to raise your heart rate and burn off extra kilojoules. You might even like to put on some lively music to boost your mood and make you go harder and faster.
- Don't sit while talking on the phone. Invest in a hands-free kit so you can walk around and be active. If you work in an office environment, why not forget the phone (or email) and actually walk to see people in the office you need to communicate with?
- Get into gardening. Jobs such as digging, weeding, raking, cutting and hauling are all good exercises, helping to build strength and stamina.

Day 17

Eat less saturated fat

WHAT IS THE IMPACT ON YOUR HEALTH?

As the Mediterranean diet has shown (being rich in olive oil, nuts, seeds and oily fish) you don't have to eat a very low-fat diet to be heart healthy. It's the type of fats you consume that can have the biggest impact on your heart. One of the main types of fat to be concerned about is saturated fats, the type usually found in animal foods such as fatty meats, cheese and butter (although they can be found in some plant foods such as coconut and palm oil). They are also common in processed foods that rely on the hardness of saturated fats (many of them are solid at room temperature) to get the right texture for baking.

Now, I like to keep things simple but it's important to explain that there are different types of saturated fat (the differences relate to their chemical structure). For example, there are short-chain, medium-chain and long-chain saturated fatty acids. The short-chain saturated fats found in coconut oil are more likely to be used as energy and less likely to be stored as fat (this is the fat found in a natural coconut not the manufactured product you buy in a tin). Even though some research has cast doubts on the strong link between saturated fats and heart disease, pointing to oxidation as the real concern, long-chain fatty acids found in beef, pork and dairy products are proven to contribute to cholesterol deposits and health problems. All oils contain varying proportions of these different fatty acids and, for the purposes of this chapter, the term 'saturated fats' will refer to all three different types as a group.

Saturated fats directly elevate your risk of heart disease by increasing LDL (bad) cholesterol levels and are primarily responsible for the sticky platelets in your blood that can form dangerous clots in your arteries.

SCIENCE SAYS

Cutting saturated fat is good for insulin control — According to the *American Institute for Cancer Research*, each percentage-point drop in saturated fat consumption generally reduces LDL (bad) by 1 to 2 per cent. They also cite research that has linked saturated fat consumption with problems in proper functioning of insulin, triggering a chain of events that leads to over-production of insulin and ultimately insulin resistance (a precursor to type 2 diabetes).

Saturated fat and central obesity — Research presented at a meeting of the American College of Cardiology found that people who eat a diet high in saturated fat accumulate more fat around the internal organs in the abdomen than those who consume healthier fats. This internal fat is also known as visceral fat and is associated with an increased risk of heart disease, high blood pressure and diabetes.

Switching dietary fats lowers cholesterol — Research published in the *European Journal of Clinical Nutrition* has shown that swapping saturated fat for either polyunsaturated or monounsaturated fats dramatically lowered cholesterol levels in a group of young adults.

Fat switch reduces risk — A study conducted at Harvard University found that replacing saturated fat-rich foods (such as meat and full-fat dairy) with foods that are rich in polyunsaturated fat (such as nuts and seeds) reduced the risk of heart disease by 19 per cent.

Type of fat, not total fat — A 2009 review of the latest research by the Heart Foundation suggests that our dietary focus should be on the type of fats we eat and not the total. They said that evidence continues to show that saturated fat leads to increased levels of LDL (bad) cholesterol in the blood, which is a major risk factor for cardiovascular disease.

PRACTICAL TIPS ON HOW TO EAT LESS SATURATED FAT

- Health authorities recommend consuming no more than 30 per cent of your total kilojoule intake from fat, of which

no more than 10 per cent should come from saturated fat.
An intake of no more than 7 per cent is recommended for
people at a high risk of heart disease.

- When you eat beef, lamb or pork, choose lean cuts over
  marbled meats; watch your portion control; and trim all
  visible fat to reduce your saturated fat intake.
- Include fish in your diet one to two times a week to help
  cut back on red meats and processed meats, which tend to
  be higher in saturated fats.
- Remove the fatty skin from chicken, turkey, duck and other
  poultry, preferably before cooking.
- Watch your intake of processed meat products such as
  ham, devon, salami, sausages, hot dogs and bacon, which
  are high in salt and saturated fat.
- Cut back on junk foods including pizza, pies, hamburgers,
  fried and battered foods, pastries and fatty snacks. Eat
  these types of food no more than once a week or preferably
  once a fortnight.
- Choose low-fat and skim dairy products such as milk,
  cheese, yoghurt and ice-cream. In some products like
  yoghurt and ice-cream, the reduced-fat content is replaced
  by sugar, so you still need to monitor your portion sizes of
  these foods.
- Use tiny servings of strongly flavoured foods like
  parmesan cheese or light sour cream to add taste when
  required.
- Cut back on the amount of butter you use on bread.
  Avocado is a healthier alternative for sandwiches.

- Avoid using butter in cooking. Replace with unsaturated oils like rice bran, olive, canola, sesame or sunflower oils.
- When having pasta or meat sauces, choose tomato-or vegetable-based options instead of creamy sauces.
- When you do have biscuits, cakes, potato crisps, corn chips or similar fatty foods keep your portions to a minimum and use the food label to help choose items with the lowest saturated fat content.

Day 18

Don't smoke, and avoid second-hand smoke

WHAT IS THE IMPACT ON YOUR HEALTH?

Cigarette smoking has a profound effect on health. There is an undeniable body of evidence to demonstrate that smoking increases the risk of death and illness from heart disease, stroke and lung cancer. Smoking constricts blood vessels, increasing the incidence of heart disease risk factors such as angina, high blood pressure and high blood cholesterol. In fact, smokers have a greater likelihood of developing at least 40 different illnesses and conditions that can reduce both quality and quantity of life, including cataracts, emphysema, osteoporosis and stomach ulcers, to name only a few. It is the number one preventable cause of death. Smokers can expect a reduction of up to 15 years in life expectancy and one out of two smokers die from their habit. Not surprisingly, there are countless health benefits from quitting. No matter how old you are or how long you've smoked, you will improve your health, fitness and appearance when you quit. Here is a timeline of some of the benefits.

- 20 minutes — Your elevated blood pressure and pulse return to normal.
- 8 hours — Increased levels of carbon monoxide and reduced levels of oxygen in your blood return to normal.
- 1 day — Your breath and clothes will smell better and you may help to improve the health of your friends, family and pets.
- 2 days — Nerve endings start to renew and your sense of smell and taste will improve. Your risk of burns and fire in and around your home is reduced.
- 2 to 12 weeks — Your circulation improves, lung function increases and exertion (such as walking up stairs) becomes easier.
- 6 months — You will experience fewer days of illness as coughing, sinus congestion, fatigue and shortness of breath decrease, and your overall level of energy improves. Your lungs begin to repair themselves, increasing the ability to handle mucus and reduce infection.
- 1 year — Your elevated risk of coronary heart disease is now half that of a smoker. Your bones have also begun to repair damage and become less brittle (and think of the money you've saved).

False security from low-tar cigarettes — A study reported in the *British Medical Journal* has shown that low-tar cigarettes offer no relief from the potential of cancer. In fact, they were responsible for a type of cancer that reaches deeper into your lung tissue.

Medical treatments help you quit — A study reported in the *British Medical Journal* has confirmed that medical treatment can help people to stop smoking. Researchers found that smokers who used nicotine gum, patches and oral medication were 22 per cent more likely to be successful at quitting after 12 months.

Passive smoking dangers for partners — Research in the *British Medical Journal* reported that exposure to second-hand smoke increases the risk of heart disease among non-smokers by as much as 60 per cent, similar to light smoking. Non-smoking women who live with smokers have up to six times more lung cancer-related chemicals in their bodies than women living with non-smokers. Partners of smokers exposed to environmental tobacco are at increased risk of lung cancer. Women whose husbands smoked in the same room had even higher levels of the cancer-linked compounds than those who smoked in a different part of the house.

Second-hand smoke reduces heart function — According to the journal *Environmental Health Perspectives*, inhaling second-hand smoke for 2 hours can cause changes in heart function that are associated with heart attack risk.

Second-hand smoke impairs blood flow — The *Journal of the American Medical Association* has reported on a study that found that even 30 minutes' exposure to second-hand smoke is enough to temporarily slow down a non-smoker's circulation. According to one of the researchers, if you sit in a smoky bar for 30 minutes, your endothelial function (the efficiency of cells that line your blood vessels) is temporarily compromised to the level of individuals who smoke a pack a day. It had a stronger impact on non-smokers than on active smokers.

Smoking increases your risk of skin cancer — According to a study published in *Nature Reviews Immunology*, skin cancer can now be added to the ever-growing list of illnesses linked to cigarette smoking. Researchers found that compared to non-smokers, people who smoke are twice as likely to develop one or more of the common types of skin cancer.

PRACTICAL TIPS ON HOW TO QUIT SMOKING

Tobacco smoke contains nicotine, an addictive drug that makes the process of quitting a challenging task. The following tips can help you deal with the cravings, withdrawal symptoms and changes to your lifestyle, increasing your chances of success.

Make a date — It is unlikely there will ever be a perfect day to quit smoking but the sooner the stop date, the better.

You can also improve your chances of giving up smoking by writing down what you need to do and how you will do it. Make a clear statement about why you are giving up cigarettes, how you will benefit and how those around you will be better off.

Seek support from friends and family — Identify the friends and family members who you think can help you to quit and enlist their support. Let them know what you are trying to achieve and how important it is to you. They can also help you to cope with situations where you may want to start smoking again.

Be prepared for temptation — After your quit date, check for events or situations that you think might entice you to start smoking. You will be tempted from time to time but you can prepare yourself by knowing your triggers, and having a plan to avoid them.

Seek medical help — If you use more than the equivalent of 10 cigarettes a day, nicotine replacement therapy can help you to reduce the withdrawal symptoms. Speak to your doctor or pharmacist about nicotine patches, gums, nasal sprays or inhalers that can help relieve the withdrawal symptoms in the early stages of quitting.

Learn from the past — The average smoker makes six to eight attempts before successfully changing or eliminating their habit. Think about when you were able to reduce or quit for a good amount of time and what helped you to succeed. Recognise and use the skills, strengths, weaknesses, resources and knowledge you already have from the past to give you options, and help you deal with the challenges in the future.

Just do it — When the day arrives it's time to become a non-smoker. Throw out any remaining tools of smoking such as all your remaining cigarettes, ashtrays, matches and lighters. Carry other things to put in your mouth such as gum, lollies, celery or carrot sticks, or a toothpick.

Change your routine — Eliminate the ties between smoking and other activities in your day-to-day life. For example, when you read the morning paper, don't sit in the same place where you used to smoke. Stay busy and plan activities to distract you when you may feel like a cigarette. Plan to exercise more and eat better as some people can gain weight after they quit.

Know how to reward yourself — Think about some small things that you enjoy such as a massage, a bath, listening to a new CD, going to the movies, reading a new book or magazine or going out to dinner. List some of these that you can use as a reward for each day or week that you remain smoke-free. You can even use the money you saved from not smoking.

Bounce back from setbacks — A slip-up or two does not mean that you have failed and is no reason to throw in the towel. Learning to stop smoking is a complex behaviour change and you may have to work on it for a while before you reach your goal. As long as you learn something positive with each quit attempt you will be further ahead next time. If you relapse, the best thing to do is to keep it small and go back to quitting as soon as you can. Look at what triggered the failure and figure out how to handle it differently next time.

Avoid passive smoke — Do your best to avoid places and situations where you will be exposed to second-hand smoke. It can trigger a relapse in a smoker who has quit and be very dangerous to the health of a non-smoker.

Day 19

Eat less trans fats

WHAT IS THE IMPACT ON YOUR HEALTH?

Trans fats, or trans fatty acids, can have a negative effect on heart health. Unlike other fats, they are not essential for our health or the provision of nutrients. While there is a category of trans fats found naturally in small amounts in some meat and dairy products (which aren't considered as harmful), they are most commonly found in processed foods as man-made fat formed by making vegetable oils into solid fats for food manufacturing. The chemical process used to solidify oil is called hydrogenation, where hydrogen gas is added to a liquid oil while it is heated under pressure. Liquid oils are hardened to make edible oil spreads to save money on manufacturing, to extend a food's shelf life and to create the desirable tastes and textures people have come to expect in processed foods. Trans fats act like saturated fats in the body but are potentially even more damaging to your health. They increase the LDL (bad) cholesterol levels and decrease healthy HDL (good) cholesterol, pushing up the risk of heart disease. Trans fats raise blood levels of triglycerides, may impair arterial flexibility and reduce insulin sensitivity, which in turn increases the risk of type 2 diabetes — a known risk factor for heart disease. What's more, whenever you eat trans fats instead of healthy fats, your antioxidant intake is less than what it could have been. It all helps to explain why countries such as Denmark have banned products containing more than 2 per cent trans fats. Since these changes were implemented in 2004, deaths from heart disease in Denmark have dropped by 20 per cent.

SCIENCE SAYS

Solid proof — There is strong evidence to support the recommendation to limit your consumption of trans fatty acids. A study reported in *The Lancet* that was carried out over 10 years found that a high intake of trans fatty acid was associated with greater risk of coronary heart disease. The study was conducted on healthy men and found those in the highest third of trans fatty acid intake had twice the risk of heart disease compared with those in the lowest third of trans fatty acid intake.

Where are your trans fats coming from? — A survey reported in the *Journal of the American Dietetic Association* found that while most respondents knew that trans fats could contribute to heart disease, less than 20 per cent could name three foods containing them. And that's in a country with strict labelling laws where trans fats must be listed.

Trans fats affect fertility — According to an eight-year study published in the *American Journal of Clinical Nutrition*, the more trans fats a woman consumes, the more likely it is she will be infertile. More specifically, for every 2 per cent increase in the amount of kilojoules a woman ate from trans fats (instead of carbohydrates), her risk of infertility went up by 73 per cent. It was estimated that this 2 per cent equates to approximately 4 grams of trans fatty acids per day. The researchers theorised that trans fats could interfere with the activity of a cell receptor involved in inflammation, glucose metabolism and insulin sensitivity, which can also impact upon heart health.

Links with depression — A six-year study published in the journal *PLoS One* found that subjects who consumed 1.5 grams of trans fats a day were 48 per cent more likely to develop depression than those who had none. According to the authors, bad fats increase inflammation, which contributes to the build-up of plaque that can cause heart disease. In the brain, substances secreted by inflammation may interfere with neurotransmitters that affect mood.

Links to colon cancer — Research published in the *American Journal of Epidemiology* found a link between the consumption of trans fats and a heightened risk of colon cancer. The study found that those who were in the top quarter of trans fat consumption had an 86 per cent higher chance of having pre-cancerous growths or polyps in their colons compared to the bottom quartile, who ate far less trans fats.

PRACTICAL TIPS ON HOW TO EAT LESS TRANS FATS

- Increase your intake of nutritious whole foods and avoid packaged and processed commercial foods.
- Get to know what foods contain this toxic fat because there is no safe level of consumption. Baked goods and the frying oils in fast foods are generally high in trans fats and are best avoided. Minimise your intake of biscuits, pies, pastries, muffins, breakfast bars, movie popcorn, cakes, fried foods (such as chicken nuggets, spring rolls, hot chips, doughnuts, fried chicken) and margarines that aren't labelled low in trans fats.
- Food manufacturers in Australia and New Zealand are not required to list trans fats on their nutrition panel unless they are making a claim about its cholesterol or fat content.
- Use the ingredients list as a guide and be wary of foods that contain 'partially hydrogenated vegetable oils' or 'hydrogenated fats'.
- Watch the spread on your bread because butter and some margarines contain trans fats. Use extra virgin olive oil instead.

Day 20

Take good care of your teeth and gums

WHAT IS THE IMPACT ON YOUR HEALTH?

Did you know that there is a strong link between the health of your gums and the health of your heart? It's thought that the bacteria that live in and around your teeth and gums can easily enter your bloodstream if you have bleeding gums. Once in your bloodstream these toxic compounds can harm the lining of your blood vessels, attaching to the fatty deposits in your arteries and increasing the risk of blood clots and heart attack.

Bleeding gums is an early symptom of gum disease, the result of plaque that builds up and separates the junction between your teeth and gums. This is also known as gingivitis. Advanced gum disease (periodontitis) is where inflammation occurs below the gum line and the gums gradually withdraw from around your teeth. Some of the common symptoms of gum disease include:

- gums that bleed easily when brushed
- red, swollen or receding gums
- bad breath
- loose teeth.

There is also a potential connection between root canal treatment and heart disease. The dead roots of a tooth treated with a root canal can become a source of chronic inflammation.

The link between gum disease and heart disease might seem obscure but the common denominator is chronic inflammation, where the build-up of plaque (different types of plaque) causes problems. Reducing inflammation is a key factor in good health, and good oral hygiene is one way to prevent chronic inflammation existing in your body. It seems that what's good for your teeth and gums is also good for the rest of your health and fitness.

SCIENCE SAYS

A clear link — Research published in the journal *Circulation* points to a clear association between gum disease and heart disease, independent of other established heart disease risk factors. Another report by the American Academy of Periodontology stated that people with gum disease are almost twice as likely to suffer coronary artery disease. It has also been linked to strokes, diabetes and low birth weights (in babies born to mothers with gum disease).

More flossing required — A study reported in the American Academy of Periodontology journal found that more than 88 per cent of people do not floss frequently enough.

Brush twice a day — A study published in the *British Medical Journal* concluded that people with the worst oral hygiene habits increased their risk of developing heart disease by 70 per cent, compared to those who brush their teeth twice a day.

Two minutes is about right — A study published in the *Journal of Clinical Periodontology* found the ideal brushing time is 2 minutes and the ideal pressure on your teeth is 150 grams, which is about the weight of an orange.

Another good reason to take care of your teeth — A study published in the *Journal of the American Dental Association* found that patients with severe heart disease or with reduced cardiac performance had more trouble bringing their heart rate and blood pressure back to normal after experiencing the stress of a dental procedure.

PRACTICAL TIPS ON HOW TO TAKE GOOD CARE OF YOUR TEETH AND GUMS

When it comes to taking care of your teeth prevention is better than cure. Good oral hygiene includes brushing, flossing, cleaning the tongue and visiting the dentist, all of which promote good dental health and prevent dental problems. The following steps can help to build and maintain strong and healthy teeth and gums, reducing your chance of developing gum disease (which may in turn help your heart).

- Brush your teeth twice a day, cleaning all surfaces of your teeth to prevent plaque build-up. Make brushing and flossing part of your routine so it becomes a habit such as just after a meal or just after a shower.
- Try to brush your teeth for around 2 minutes, focusing on the benefits of clean healthy teeth, not the time it takes you to clean them.
- Use a soft-bristled toothbrush angled at 45 degrees and perform short, circular motions to clean the junction between your teeth and gums. Brush with a light amount of pressure.
- Try to focus on quality brushing rather than quantity. Brushing your teeth too hard or for too long can cause more harm than good by damaging the tooth enamel and gums.
- An electric toothbrush is a good investment and has a greater chance of removing more plaque after 2 minutes of brushing.
- Try to floss your teeth at least once a day to remove the plaque build-up from between your teeth where brushing can't reach. This prevents decay and can help keep your breath fresh.
- Eat a healthy diet low in processed foods, especially foods and drinks containing sugar. Pay extra attention to oral hygiene if you snack on sugary foods between meals or if you have a sweet tooth. By avoiding sugar you prevent the development of bacteria that cause plaque build-up.

- If you don't have the opportunity to brush your teeth after a sugary snack, rinse your mouth out with water.
- Use a good fluoride toothpaste.
- Replace your brush every three to four months or when the bristles become frayed or curly.
- See your dentist and hygienist regularly. Dentists and hygienists can screen for heart disease, which has oral symptoms. Dentists may even detect medical conditions in their early stages if they see patients on a regular basis.
- If you consistently have bleeding gums, visit your dentist and have them help you to review your oral hygiene practices.

Day 21

Drink enough water

WHAT IS THE IMPACT ON YOUR HEALTH?

It's often said that we should drink six to eight glasses of water every day simply for good health. But when you stop to think about the impact that water intake has on your heart, it makes sense. Ultimately the level of water in your body helps determine the viscosity of your blood. Thinner blood puts less stress on your heart, while thicker blood increases blood pressure and the concentration of blood-clotting agents. Water is absorbed quickly and easily into the bloodstream and thins the blood, helping to prevent artery-clogging clots. Therefore, drinking plenty of water and staying consistently hydrated can potentially protect your heart and reduce the risk of heart attack. It could be just as important to your heart as healthy eating, regular exercise and avoiding tobacco. Water has even been described as the unexpected blood pressure drug, with the additional benefit that it can be consumed at minimal cost and is without side effects. But this benefit only comes from drinking plain water (tap or bottled).

The consumption of other fluids, including juice, soft drink, milk and alcohol does not offer the same protective benefits. These beverages all require digestion and may cause fluids to move from the blood into the gut, which could potentially thicken the blood. However, tea and alcohol may offer some additional heart health benefits, although a number of conditions apply in terms of how they are consumed (see Day 34 for details).

A secondary heart health benefit of drinking enough water when compared to other kilojoule-laden fluids is that it can help manage your weight. Conversely, mild dehydration is a common cause of constipation and daytime sleepiness.

SCIENCE SAYS

Don't become dehydrated — According to the *American Journal of Epidemiology*, chronic dehydration can increase the risk of high blood pressure, atherosclerosis and coronary heart disease.

Drink at least five glasses — A study reported in the *American Journal of Epidemiology* conducted on over 20,000 subjects found that people who drank five or more glasses of water each day had only half the risk of fatal heart disease compared with those who drank two or fewer glasses per day.

Secondary heart benefit (weight loss) — A study reported in the *Journal of the American Dietetic Association* showed that drinking 500 millilitres of water 30 minutes before a meal can help to reduce the kilojoule intake of that meal. In addition, a study reported in the *Journal of Pediatrics* found that kids who drank water instead of juice and soft drinks reduced their risk of being overweight by an amazing 31 per cent.

Metabolism bonus — According to the *American Journal of Physiology*, drinking cold water can result in a small elevation in your metabolic rate, which may help to boost fat loss.

Dehydration can lead to salt preference — Research reported in the journal *Medical Hypotheses* found that previous experiences of dehydration seem to lead individuals to a preference for salt. Because of the negative effect salt can have on your blood pressure, this is another reason to try and stay hydrated.

PRACTICAL TIPS ON HOW TO DRINK ENOUGH WATER

- Your body loses approximately 2 litres of water every day through urine, sweat, your breath and bowel movements. So you need to replace that lost fluid for your body to function to its best potential.
- Kilojoule-free water is the best choice for your heart, your weight and your health. Water thins the blood, while other fluids draw water out of the blood to aid in their digestion. It's important to recognise that there is a difference for

heart health between getting fluids from plain water and from fruit juice.

- There is no 'one size fits all' rule on how much water to drink. This is because water needs vary considerably between individuals — and according to circumstances — due to weight, age, gender, diet and other beverages consumed, air temperature and humidity, occupation, fitness and physical activity levels, illness, even clothing and the type of material it is made out of.
- One helpful guide is to drink 30 millilitres of water per kilogram of body weight every day. For example, a 70-kilogram person would need to drink 2100 millilitres of water a day or just over 2 litres.
- Try drinking one to two glasses of water before meals. The extra fullness may also help to reduce your portion sizes, which can assist with weight management.
- Drink water to quench your thirst. Only drink other kilojoule-laden beverages in small amounts for taste.
- Don't wait to feel thirsty. Try to make drinking water a habit by adding it on to other habits such as before eating, after going to the toilet or after brushing your teeth.
- Drink a little extra water if it's hot or if you work in an air-conditioned office.
- Exercise increases your need for fluids above and beyond your normal daily needs. Unless your activity lasts for longer than 90 minutes, sports drinks are unnecessary. Consume 150 to 200 millilitres of water for 15 to 20 minutes of exercise.

- Have a water bottle on hand at your desk, in your fridge and in your car.
- Be more aware of your water intake as you get older. Between the ages of 60 and 70, people start to lose their appetite and consequently get less water from foods in their diet.
- If you take medications that have a diuretic effect or if you use fibre tablets, include an extra glass of water each day.
- If you don't like water straight up, add a slice of lemon, lime or orange.
- Don't keep juice, soft drink or cordial in your house. If it's hard to get you'll be less likely to have it.
- Give your tastebuds time to adjust to drinking fewer sugar-laden drinks. As with cutting sugar out of your tea or coffee, you will get used to it after a while.
- Solid food does contribute to your total fluid needs, especially plant foods such as fruits and vegetables, which should be a focus of your diet.
- The digestion of protein requires extra water. If you are on a high-protein diet or if you consume protein supplements, increase your water intake proportionately.
- You can also get too much of a good thing. Over-hydration occurs when you drink more water than the kidneys and liver can process in one day, resulting in nausea and the leaching of important nutrients.

Day 22

Moderate your salt intake

WHAT IS THE IMPACT ON YOUR HEALTH?

Salt may also be referred to as sodium but there is a difference. Sodium is an ingredient in salt because other things are also added to table salt such as anti-caking agents. For the purposes of this tip I will use the less scientific term 'salt', but I am also referring to sodium.

Salt is sometimes referred to as 'white death' due to its strong association with an increased risk of high blood pressure, heart disease and stroke. According to the World Health Organization, high blood pressure is the world's third leading cause of death and disability. Too much salt can also raise your risk of kidney stones, stomach cancer and osteoporosis. Salt helps regulate the balance of water in the body (among other functions). Excess salt in our diet pushes up the salt content in the blood. This triggers the kidneys to retain more water in our blood vessels in an attempt to keep the salt concentration balanced. The extra water in your arteries increases pressure, resulting in higher blood pressure. Conversely, the mineral potassium (found in whole foods such as fruits and vegetables) helps reduce blood pressure by keeping blood vessel walls relaxed.

SCIENCE SAYS

Less salt is good for your bones — Researchers at the University of Western Australia found post-menopausal women who reduced their salt intake minimised the loss of calcium from their bones. A reduction in salt gave as much bone protection as adding 1000 milligrams of calcium to the diet.

Less salt equals lower blood pressure — A scientific trial reported in the *Journal of Human Hypertension* compared two groups of moderately overweight, middle-aged adults with pre-hypertension. After three years, those who cut their salt intake by 25 per cent (by roughly 930 milligrams per day) had blood pressure readings that were lower than those who didn't eat less salt.

Less salt even helps if you don't have high blood pressure — A study reported in the *Annals of Internal Medicine* found that a low-fat diet full of fruits and vegetables but little salt can lead to a significant drop in blood pressure, even in people with normal blood pressure.

Salt may affect people differently — According to

Hypertension, the journal of the American Heart Association, genetic variations influence which patients with hypertension will experience a reduction in blood pressure following dietary salt restriction. The researchers stated that until we understand more, anyone with high blood pressure should reduce their salt intake.

Double dose — It has been estimated that Australians eat an average of 9 grams of salt each day, more than twice the daily suggested dietary intake of 4 grams (or 1600 milligrams of salt). In reality, we could happily survive on 1 to 2 grams per day. While we do need some salt in our diet there is enough present naturally in whole foods. It's estimated that a dietary reduction of 3 grams of salt per day per person would prevent between 3000 and 6000 deaths in Australia each year.

Less salt is helpful for women — The *Journal of the American College of Cardiology* found that cutting back on salt was even more effective at lowering blood pressure than exercising. The three-month study found that the average drop in systolic pressure (the higher number) for women who limited their salt intake to 2.4 grams was about 16 mmHg, compared with 5 mmHg among those who walked for 30 minutes on three to four days each week.

Go easy on cheese, processed meat and sauces — Australian research reported in 2010 in the *American Journal of Clinical Nutrition* found that over 70 per cent of processed meats, cheeses and sauces (especially Asian sauces such as fish, oyster and soy) contain unacceptably high salt levels.

Activity reduces the impact of salt on blood pressure According to the American Heart Association, exercise may help to prevent salt from elevating blood pressure levels. People who exercised the most in the study had a 38 per cent lower risk of being sensitive to a high-salt diet compared with people who didn't exercise at all. According to the researchers, the more exercise you do, the less of an effect salt may have on your blood pressure.

Having less salt is on a par with taking blood pressure-lowering drugs — *The New England Journal of Medicine* has reported on findings of a study showing cutting back on salt and eating more fruits, vegetables and low-fat dairy products can reduce blood pressure to a level equal with that achieved by blood pressure-lowering medication. People in this study consumed no more than 1500 milligrams of salt daily.

Reduce your risk — A report by the *British Medical Journal* found that cutting down your salt intake by a third could result in a 23 per cent reduction in stroke and a 14 per cent decrease in heart disease. This reduction in risk was significant because it occurred in people who didn't have high blood pressure. In other words, reducing your salt intake may be beneficial for more reasons than just reduced blood pressure.

PRACTICAL TIPS ON HOW TO MODERATE YOUR SALT INTAKE

- Get to know how much salt is in the foods you commonly eat. You might be surprised how much salt is in some everyday foods such as breakfast cereals, bread, biscuits and sauces. Other foods to be wary of include soup, packet pasta or noodles, canned fish, pizza, hamburgers, marinades, lunch meats (ham) and processed meats like sausages and salami.

- Roast your own meats at home (such as pork, chicken, beef or lamb) for use on sandwiches instead of processed meats. Lunch meats such as ham are very high in salt.

- A lot of the salt consumed in our diet is hidden in foods not even thought of as salty such as bread and breakfast cereals. Many of us eat too much salt without even shaking it over a meal or adding it during food preparation. Only a small percentage (between 10 and 20 per cent) of the salt we consume is thought to come out of the table salt shaker. While it is advisable to avoid adding salt to your food, or to do so in small amounts, cutting out table salt will not be enough on its own to significantly cut back your salt intake.

- Cut back on processed foods, packaged foods, pre-prepared meals and takeaway. Eat more whole foods with one single ingredient such as vegetables and fruit (which contain potassium), oats, fish, legumes and unsalted nuts and seeds, and very little salt.

- Be wary of snack foods that are high in salt such as crackers, savoury biscuits, potato crisps, pretzels and salted nuts.

- You need to be a good label reader to reduce your salt intake. Salt is listed as sodium on the nutrition information panels on food labels, which you can use to compare similar items and choose foods with as little salt as possible. Foods with less than 120 milligrams of sodium per 100 grams are considered low in salt, while those which contain more than 480 milligrams of sodium per 100 grams are considered high in salt. It helps to shop around. One Australian survey found 100 times more salt in one variety of canned tomatoes compared to another.
- When looking at the ingredients list on food labels get to know the alternative names for salt, including sodium bicarbonate, stock cubes, baking powder, yeast extract, monosodium glutamate and rock salt.
- Look for the 'Low Salt' or 'No Added Salt' option when choosing canned foods and sauces.
- Our tastebuds become less sensitive over time and there may be a tendency to add more salt, even though blood pressure can actually increase with age. This is all the more reason to be aware of your salt intake as you get older and work at finding ways to add flavour to your foods without salt.
- Look to other low-salt alternatives to add flavour to your foods. Some suggestions include garlic, lemon juice, herbs and spices. Keep in mind that spice mixes can have added salt.
- Try to eat no more than 4 grams of salt (or 1600 milligrams of sodium) each day. This equates to approximately one teaspoon of salt.

- The salt content of fast food is generally very high. Check company websites and even nutrition information, which is sometimes provided. Fast food is certainly something that should be consumed rarely if you want to reduce your salt intake.
- It's not just the fast-food restaurants that are liberal in their use of salt. The salt content of meals at fine dining and sit-down restaurants can also be high. Ask for sauces on the side and ask the waiter for low-salt options.
- As far as your heart is concerned there is no significant difference between table salt and sea salt. They may be produced differently, but they both contain sodium and your health will benefit from avoiding both types of salt.
- You can also buy iodised versions of salt, which is table salt mixed with a minute amount of iodine. Iodine deficiency has an impact on mental and thyroid health, and iodised salt provides a small but essential amount for people who need it. Iodine also occurs naturally in seafood, vegetables, meat, eggs, dairy products and grain-based foods.
- Give your tastebuds time to adjust to eating less salt. While it may take four to six weeks, your heart will benefit for it.

Day 23

Get your anger under control

WHAT IS THE IMPACT ON YOUR HEALTH?

When well managed, anger or irritation has very few detrimental health or interpersonal consequences. But when anger gets out of control it can alienate family, friends and co-workers, becoming a very destructive emotion both socially and physically. It can be triggered by pain, frustration or disappointment and can range from a slight annoyance to hostility and rage. One person can experience anger very differently from the next, including:

- How easily they get angry.
- How intensely anger is felt.
- How long it lasts.
- How often anger occurs.
- How they express their anger.

Anger can have a detrimental effect on your health, triggering the release of chemicals such as catecholamines, the compounds that constrict blood vessels, increase heart rate and raise blood pressure. Men and women who are known to be more hostile than most people are also likely to have higher levels of homocysteine, a blood chemical strongly associated with coronary heart disease. Elevated levels of homocysteine are thought to cause damage to the cells lining the walls of arteries, which contributes to the development of arterial plaque.

SCIENCE SAYS

Anger increases heart risk — A study published in the journal *Annals of Family Medicine* has shown that middle-aged men who have high levels of anger are more at risk of developing heart disease than calm men. Men with high trait anger scores were 1.7 times more likely to develop high blood pressure compared to men with low or moderate scores.

Get a grip on gripe sessions — According to the *Archives of Internal Medicine*, men who reported that they became irritable, expressed their anger, felt angry but concealed the emotion and participated in gripe sessions had a higher risk of premature heart disease and heart attack. This was compared with men who were less angry, and was independent of other variables such as cholesterol levels, body mass index (BMI) and blood pressure.

Exercise provides a protective effect against anger — A study reported in the *Journal of Behavioral Medicine* found that women prone to angry outbursts had less healthy cholesterol levels than their calmer peers. However, women who were angry but physically fit showed no such ill effects on their cholesterol levels. This also reflects earlier findings in men where fitness was also shown to counter the negative cardiovascular effects of anger.

Men more likely to be hostile — A study published in the journal *Life Sciences* found that men had higher levels of hostility and inhibition of anger compared to women.

Mind your temper — Research reported in the *Archives of Internal Medicine* found that hot-tempered men are more likely to develop premature heart disease and suffer an early heart attack compared with their more relaxed peers. Men who responded to stressful situations with feelings of anger and irritability were three times more likely to be diagnosed with heart disease, and five times as likely to have a heart attack before the age of 55.

Good nutrition and supplements — A study reported in the *British Journal of Psychiatry* found that prisoners given supplements containing vitamins, minerals and essential fatty acids showed a reduction in violence and antisocial behaviour compared to prisoners taking a placebo (or sugar pill). The researchers believe that the effect of diet on antisocial behaviour has been underestimated.

Angry women at higher risk — According to the journal *Psychosomatic Medicine*, women who harbour feelings of anger or depression are more likely to have heart disease risk factors such as high cholesterol and an unhealthy weight. Women rated as the most hostile had the highest levels of LDL (bad) cholesterol and the lowest levels of HDL (good) cholesterol.

Anger may lead to atrial fibrillation — According to a study published in the journal *Circulation*, men who described themselves as fiery (or quick-tempered), hot-headed, furious when criticised or wanting to hit someone when frustrated were 30 per cent more likely to suffer from atrial fibrillation, an irregular heart rhythm that can lead to sudden death.

PRACTICAL TIPS ON HOW TO KEEP YOUR ANGER UNDER CONTROL

Treating anger can help to improve your quality of life and may help to slow the progression of heart-related illness. Learning how to constructively deal with anger has the potential to benefit your physical and emotional health. Consider the following strategies to help keep your anger under control.

- When you start to feel angry, practise deep breathing exercises and positive self-talk.
- Keep a log of moments when you feel anger or have angry outbursts to increase your awareness of the circumstances that make you angry.

- If you are prone to anger, getting enough regular exercise is a priority for your heart health.
- Seek out suitable ways to express your anger such as boxing classes, tennis or golf.
- Find someone you can talk to rather than bottling up any anger inside. Learning to express your feelings calmly and rationally may help to keep at bay any hostility.
- As you seek to gain greater control over anger be aware that there may be an inclination to rely on alcohol and other drugs as a source of relief. Try to make a list of activities and pursuits that help you unwind and relax that aren't detrimental to your health.
- If you believe your anger is out of control you could seek the help of a mental health professional or look for an anger management class in your local area.

Day 24

Get more antioxidants in your diet

WHAT IS THE IMPACT ON YOUR HEALTH?

There is a constant battle going on within your body between antioxidants and free radicals. As the name states, antioxidants are compounds that prevent oxygen damage (oxidation) and fight the action of free radicals. Free radicals are unstable oxygen molecules missing an electron and they damage other cells by seeking out a full complement of electrons. By taking electrons from otherwise healthy cells, the damage they cause (oxidation) can accumulate, partly contributing to the ageing process and the development of heart disease and some cancers. For example, the oxidation of LDL (bad) cholesterol is associated with the hardening of arteries that can lead to heart disease. Free radicals are formed within our bodies as a natural by-product of metabolism and even exercise. Some free radicals are even helpful in the fight against infection and bacteria. But too many can be damaging, especially free radicals from external sources such as ultraviolet radiation, pollution and cigarette smoke.

Antioxidants such as vitamins C, E and beta-carotene may play a preventative role in ageing and the development of heart disease by neutralising free radicals. Antioxidants 'donate' electrons to free radicals, rendering them non-reactive and less likely to have a negative impact on other cells.

To help better understand the action of free radicals and antioxidants, think about how a sliced apple turns brown. The inner flesh is exposed to air, allowing oxygen to create cell damage, but if you drizzle some fresh lemon juice over the sliced apple the browning does not occur. The vitamin C (a potent antioxidant) in the lemon inhibits oxidation and prevents cellular damage.

SCIENCE SAYS

Olive oil is rich in antioxidants — Research published in the *Federation of American Societies for Experimental Biology Journal* showed that olive oil contains a number of compounds called phenols, which are believed to act as powerful antioxidants that may help prevent cancer. People who consume plenty of olive oil may be helping to prevent damage to their body cells that can eventually lead to cancer. It may also help explain why certain cancers, including breast, colon, ovarian and prostate cancers, are less common in Mediterranean countries.

Go for food over supplements — There are a number of contradictory studies regarding the use of supplemental antioxidants. Until a greater body of evidence is established, the best source of antioxidants is through a healthy diet. After all, supplements can't help you overcome bad diet.

Lutein is a sight for sore eyes — Lutein, an antioxidant nutrient already linked to eye health, may help prevent the hardening and narrowing of arteries that can lead to heart attack and stroke, according to a report in *Circulation*, the journal of the American Heart Association. Researchers found that subjects with the highest blood levels of lutein showed the least thickening in their artery walls over 18 months. Lutein-rich foods include dark leafy greens, orange juice, carrots and eggs.

Vitamin C for blood flow — According to research found in the *Journal of the American Diabetes Association*, obese subjects who were given vitamin C experienced a widening of their blood vessels and improved blood flow. The researchers also cited previous research which found that antioxidant vitamins such as C and E may help arteries dilate and keep blood flowing smoothly.

A boost for men's health — According to a recent study published in the *Journal of Nutrition*, antioxidants may significantly reduce the risk of developing lower urinary tract symptoms in men. The antioxidants in this study were from dietary not supplemental sources.

PRACTICAL TIPS ON HOW TO INCLUDE MORE ANTIOXIDANTS IN YOUR DIET

There are many different types of antioxidants and the best approach is to include a broad range of plant-based foods in your diet. Use the following guidelines to help boost the antioxidant content of your diet.

- Eat plenty of fresh foods every day. By eating lots of fruits and vegetables every day, your body will have a constant supply of molecules that may help neutralise free radicals. Aim for at least five servings of vegetables and two servings of fruit.
- By eating an assortment of different coloured fruits and vegetables, you increase your exposure to a wide variety of nutrients. Vibrant colours may correspond with more vitamins and antioxidants; experiment with red, green, orange, yellow and blue fruits and vegetables.
- Include yellow and orange fruits and vegetables such as carrots, sweet potato, orange and yellow capsicum, corn, peaches, apricots, oranges and rockmelon. These are good sources of the antioxidant beta-carotene, the plant form of vitamin A.
- Include dark green leafy vegetables such as spinach, broccoli, cabbage, kale and salad greens like lettuce for a variety of antioxidants, including vitamins E and C and beta-carotene.

- Include citrus fruits and red fruits and vegetables such as oranges, mandarins and lemon, along with red capsicum, tomatoes, red grapes, strawberries and raspberries, which are rich sources of the antioxidant vitamin C.
- Include in your diet some plant and seafood fats such as nuts, seeds, avocado, olive oil and vegetable oils that are high in the antioxidant vitamin E. Fish and seafood also contain vitamin E.
- Use healthy cooking methods such as steaming, microwaving, grilling or stir frying, which minimise the loss of nutrients, and opt for minimal cooking times for vegetables.
- Expand your fruit and vegetable horizons by experimenting with varieties that you haven't used before or have used infrequently. Be adventurous.

Day 25

Get enough sleep

WHAT IS THE IMPACT ON YOUR HEALTH?

There is a very strong relationship between sleep and health, and many of us are not getting enough. It's thought that blood pressure tends to fall off during sleep, protecting your heart. Sleep deprivation, however, causes your blood vessels to constrict and may actually increase blood pressure.

Another possibility is that long-term sleep deprivation might inflame the linings of the arteries. Just a few nights of sleep loss has been shown to raise the level of inflammation markers.

Sleep may also protect your health by reducing the release of the stress hormone cortisol. In fact, too little sleep can alter the balance of several hormones which, in turn, can increase appetite and negatively impact upon your insulin resistance, immune function and metabolic rate. Insulin resistance means your body uses more insulin to keep your blood sugar where it should be and high insulin levels are a major contributor to fat storage and vascular disease. What's more, a slower metabolic rate can reduce your body's capacity to burn kilojoules, which can trigger weight gain and increase your risk of heart disease. People who are tired get hungry and tend to eat more in an attempt to boost their energy levels.

Another problem with a lack of sleep is that it makes you feel fatigued, making it harder to motivate yourself to exercise or cook healthy meals. Sustained, unbroken sleep is an important way to recharge your body and mind, and help your body function at its best. By waking up fresh and alert, you'll be more likely to feel like exercise and you can face the day with a positive outlook. Adequate sleep can rank equally with a healthy diet and regular exercise as a crucial part of a healthy lifestyle.

SCIENCE SAYS

Seven might be the magic number — People who sleep for either more or fewer than 7 hours a day, including naps, have an increased risk of cardiovascular disease.

Get more than 5 hours (women) — A 2002 review of the Nurses' Health Study (on over 70,000 women) found that women who slept less than 5 hours a night had a 32 per cent greater risk of heart disease compared to women who had 8 hours sleep. These figures also took into account other lifestyle factors that can increase heart disease risk such as diabetes, snoring, high blood pressure, depression, shift work, alcohol use and smoking.

Nine or more may be too much — The same Nurses' Health Study found that sleeping too much may also have a detrimental effect on heart health. People who slept 9 or more hours also had more heart attacks, though there was not as big an effect. It's possible that people who slept this long had some kind of sleep disorder that was associated with other medical problems.

Get more than 5 hours (men) — Men who frequently work long hours or get little sleep are at twice the risk of suffering a non-fatal heart attack, researchers have found. The heightened risk occurred in men who slept for 5 hours or less (on average) each working day during the previous year compared with men who got more than 5 hours of sleep nightly. The findings were published in the journal *Occupational and Environmental Medicine*.

Get an extra hour — Just 1 extra hour of sleep a day appears to lower the risk of developing calcium deposits in the arteries, a known risk factor for heart disease. Every additional hour that people slept, their risk of having a coronary calcification went down by a third. Of the subjects who had slept less than 5 hours a night, 27 per cent had developed artery calcification after five years. That dropped to 11 per cent among those who slept 5 to 7 hours, and to 6 per cent among those who slept more than

7 hours a night. The findings were reported in the *Journal of the American Medical Association*.

Stay lean — A study reported in the *Journal of Physiology* on 24 pairs of identical twins found that the fatter of each pair had a worse sleep pattern and was more likely to snore than his or her lean sibling. It seems that one of the first areas of the body to store excess fat is the tongue and throat, resulting in airway restriction and snoring. In advanced cases, excess body fat can increase the risk of sleep apnoea. This also restricts the intake of oxygen and disturbs deep sleep as the body wakes itself up to restore normal breathing. Along with an increased risk of heart disease, sleep apnoea can result in fatigue and excessive daytime sleepiness. It seems that both heart health and sleep quality can be improved by reducing body fat.

PRACTICAL TIPS ON HOW TO GET ENOUGH SLEEP

- Go to bed and, even more importantly, get up at the same time every day. Establishing a routine can make a big difference to your sleep quality. Try to avoid sleeping in on weekends.
- Make your preparation for sleep a priority. Have a pre-sleep ritual such as dimming the lights, having a bath or shower, reading or listening to quiet music. You could even try some deep breathing exercises.
- Make sure your room is dark. Even small amounts of light at night can interfere with sleep quality. Darkness triggers the release of hormones that help you fall asleep.

- Create the right environment for sleep. Make sure your room is free from noise and distractions. You will also sleep better if your room is well ventilated and kept at a cool, comfortable temperature.
- Avoid large, spicy meals, cigarettes, alcohol and caffeine close to bedtime. These can all make it harder to fall asleep, or reduce your quality of sleep.
- Be physically active during the day to help you fall asleep at night. Avoid exercise at night if you have trouble falling asleep.
- Napping is beneficial if you are chronically sleep deprived (such as shift workers), but it can interfere with your night-time sleep. Try to avoid napping unless you've had less than 5 to 6 hours sleep.
- Avoid sleeping pills. They are not a long-term solution for poor sleeping habits.
- Learn to reduce thinking and worrying in bed. To help put your mind at ease plan out your next day before you go to bed. Find ways to unwind and manage your stress.
- Make changes to your sleep routine gradually. Just like any lifestyle habit, give yourself a little time to adapt to these changes, and don't try to change too much too soon.

Day 26

Eat more garlic

WHAT IS THE IMPACT ON YOUR HEALTH?

Garlic's health benefits are well known. It has a good reputation for preventing colds and flu, and there is evidence to suggest that it can provide a range of heart health benefits. It's thought garlic may help to support healthy blood flow, normalise blood pressure and decrease elevated levels of cholesterol in the blood, although some of the research is inconclusive (see 'Science says' below for more details).

Garlic is rich in manganese, vitamins B6, B1 and C, and protein. Garlic has a number of sulphur-containing compounds which are thought to give it its characteristic smell. One of these compounds, allicin, is also thought to be an antioxidant and partially responsible for garlic's anti-viral and lipid-lowering properties.

Another heart benefit comes from the fact that garlic is thought to help the body fight inflammation and may help lower homocysteine levels. Garlic is also a potential fat fighter because it is lipotropic, which means it helps catalyse the breakdown of fat during metabolism in the body.

SCIENCE SAYS

Cholesterol lowering — According to *The Journal of the Royal College of Physicians*, test subjects taking garlic experienced a 12 per cent reduction in total cholesterol in only four weeks compared to subjects taking a placebo. Triglycerides (a measure of fat in blood) also dropped by 17 per cent compared to the placebo group.

Capsules are also beneficial — A study reported in Penn State's College of Health and Human Development found that deodorised garlic capsules helped bring down men's blood cholesterol levels by 7 per cent over five months. Men taking a placebo capsule had no change in their cholesterol levels.

Conflicting research on cholesterol — A comprehensive study reported in the *Archives of Internal Medicine* found that raw garlic and two popular garlic supplements had only a small effect on cholesterol levels after subjects consumed the equivalent of four cloves per day, six days a week for six months. It seems that garlic's impact on cholesterol may be small, although it also offers additional antioxidant benefits which may help to prevent atherosclerosis.

Atherosclerosis assistance — According to a study published in the journal *Life Sciences*, consuming 1 millilitre of a garlic extract per kilogram of body weight for six months resulted in a significant reduction in oxidant (free radical) stress in the blood of arteriosclerosis patients.

Garlic is good for blood thinning — A study conducted at Saarland University in Germany found that compounds present in garlic help blood clots to dissolve more quickly, improving the fluidity of blood.

Garlic is relaxing for your blood vessels — A study published in the *Proceedings of the National Academy of Sciences* claims to have found the reason why garlic offers so many health benefits. Eating a diet rich in garlic increases the production of hydrogen sulfide in your blood, which relaxes your blood vessels and elevates blood flow, protecting your heart and preventing some cancers.

Cancer cutter — A study published in the *Journal of Nutrition* found that the more raw and cooked garlic the participants of the study consumed, the lower their risk of stomach and colorectal cancer.

Bowel health bonus — According to research presented in *New Scientist* magazine, there are potential bowel cancer reducing benefits by eating as little as half a clove of garlic a day. However, the authors did state that the garlic was raw and that you'd need to eat four cloves of cooked garlic to get the same benefits.

Men's health bonus — Research published in the *Journal of the National Cancer Institute* found that a high consumption (at least 10 grams per day) of allium vegetables, such as garlic, was associated with a 50 per cent decrease in the risk of prostate cancer.

An even bigger bonus for men's health — A small study conducted at the St Thomas Hospital in London found that six out of seven men experienced an improvement in their erectile function after eating four cloves of garlic a day for three months.

PRACTICAL TIPS ON HOW TO EAT MORE GARLIC

- There are a number of ways you can include more garlic in your diet. Garlic comes in many forms, including fresh, minced, capsule, powdered or as an oil.

- Minced garlic (that comes in a jar) makes it easier to add garlic to meals. It's made up of approximately 96 per cent garlic, so it's only a small trade-off for convenience when it's always available quickly and easily in your fridge. One teaspoon of minced garlic is equivalent to approximately one bulb of garlic.

- Add garlic to a wide variety of savoury meals such as soups, casseroles, scrambled eggs, stir-fries, cooked vegetables and pasta sauces.

- Because much of the research is conflicting, don't rely on garlic alone to help reduce your cholesterol levels. But even if future research eventually proves that garlic has no impact on cholesterol levels it still has a number of health-giving properties. And it's a tasty alternative to salt.

- The most notable side effect from eating garlic is the presence of odour on your breath. To combat this have a little chopped fresh parsley after your garlic indulgence.
- It's thought that garlic may interact with blood-thinning medications such as warfarin. If you have any concerns, discuss them with your doctor.
- Garlic is fantastic roasted. Preheat the oven to 180°C, and place the cloves (skin and all) in the oven for 20 minutes or until soft. The skins should peel off easily and the garlic can be eaten with other roasted vegetables, spread over toast or used in a dip with mashed cannellini beans and chopped parsley. Yum!
- Many studies into garlic talk about eating two to four cloves a day to obtain health benefits but this may seem like a lot to some people. Aim for half to one clove a day initially, building up your intake gradually.

Day 27

Be in a relationship and work together for improved health

WHAT IS THE IMPACT ON YOUR HEALTH?

Being in a relationship has a wide range of health benefits, with research showing there is a clear link between marriage and better health. A lot of the known health benefits are based on research on married couples but it would be fair to assume these benefits apply to anyone in a committed, long-term relationship. Happy couples are known to have a number of physical and emotional advantages over their single counterparts, including a longer life, more satisfying sexual relationships, improved mental health, a reduced risk of drug and alcohol abuse, fewer sexually transmitted diseases and lower rates of suicide. The simple act of living with someone can be good for your health, with the potential for better care in times of emergency or illness. Happy couples are also more likely to nurture and look out for each other by promoting a good diet and a healthy lifestyle. Working together with your partner on the road to health and wellness can make the journey a whole lot easier. The support and understanding that only a partner can give provides couples with a unique opportunity to share the journey towards a healthy heart, even a better relationship. After all, nobody else has a better insight into your attitude, habits, strengths and weaknesses. But just as a good marriage is associated with health benefits, a bad marriage can have negative health consequences, with evidence to suggest that marital disharmony is a risk factor for illness and disease.

SCIENCE SAYS

Partner assistance — A study published in the *American Journal of Health Studies* found that your exercise routine will be more likely to stay on track by involving your partner. A study that examined the dropout rates at gyms found that couples who joined together were six times more likely to still be exercising 12 months later than married people who joined alone.

Married men live longer — The Australian Bureau of Statistics reported in 2006 that married men live longer than lifelong single men. Additional research published in *BMC Public Health* reported similar findings, where never married men had a significantly higher risk of death from all causes compared to married men.

Stroke risk for single or unhappy men — A study reported on by the American Stroke Association found that single men and men who were unsatisfied with their marriage had a 64 per cent higher risk of fatal stroke than happily married men. Unhappy men are prone to overeating, exercising less, drinking more and smoking and are less likely to have health checks or take medication. This leads to increased weight, high blood pressure and elevated cholesterol, all of which increase the risk of stroke and heart disease.

Old wounds may not heal — A 2005 study published in the *Archives of General Psychiatry* found a connection between marital conflict and impaired wound healing. Couples who were classified as highly hostile had greater levels of pro-inflammatory cytokines in their blood, which resulted in slower wound healing compared to low-level hostile couples. Sustained elevated levels of pro-inflammatory cytokines have been linked with a wide range of age-related diseases and may enhance the development of depressive symptoms.

Love is good for the heart — According to the World Heart Federation, love is good for our hearts, helping to reduce stress, depression and anxiety, which are all major risk factors for heart disease. They quoted a five-year study where 10,000 men at high risk of developing heart disease-related chest pain (angina) were asked, 'Does your wife show you her love?' Those who said 'Yes' had half the risk of getting angina.

Love and support are helpful after heart attack — A study published in the British Medical Association's journal, *Heart*, found that heart attack survivors with a close friend, relative or lover to confide in are half as likely to suffer further heart attacks within a year as patients without a shoulder to cry on.

Be romantic and recite poetry — According to the *International Journal of Cardiology*, there is a significant stress-releasing effect from the recitation of poetry. The subjects who recited poetry for 30 minutes had a slower heart and breathing rate and experienced a level of deep relaxation afterwards compared to subjects engaged in conversation for 30 minutes.

PRACTICAL TIPS ON HOW TO MAKE YOUR RELATIONSHIP A HEALTHY AND HAPPY ONE

By joining forces you can help each other move more, eat better, and stay positive about lifestyle changes. By motivating and encouraging each other you can also have fun working together towards a common interest. Use the following tips to boost the health of your heart and your relationship.

- Set a good example. You won't motivate your partner to exercise more by lying on the couch. By setting a healthy example your partner will see how it's possible to make healthy changes with a similar lifestyle. Make improvements to your own eating and exercise habits and be a positive role model.

- Identify obstacles and solutions. Talk to each other about the things that hold you back from exercising more or eating better. If you identify one of your partner's limiting factors, do so in a positive way. Whether it's too much alcohol on weekends or too much chocolate in front of the television, don't nag your partner about their faults. Be constructive and offer solutions that the two of you can work on together.

- Have a plan. Make a note of the physical activity you intend to do on a weekly basis and what activities will potentially involve your partner. Whether it's a game of tennis on Thursday night or a bushwalk on Sunday morning, planning ahead will make it more likely to happen. You don't have to do something together every day or even have the same health and fitness goals, but let your partner be aware of your plan so they can support and encourage you.

- Just do it — together. A little teamwork can go a long way. Prioritise the time you spend exercising with your partner or preparing a healthy meal together. If you have different schedules, alternate nights where you cook a lean and tasty feast for each other. Try shopping together to prevent fatty treats finding their way into your trolley and go for an evening stroll to unwind rather than watching television.

- Share the rewards. Give yourselves an incentive for sticking with your plan for a set period of time. If you've had a good month, reward yourselves with a massage or trip to the movies. You can even work towards greater rewards when you achieve your goals, such as a holiday or new treadmill. Just avoid food-based rewards that undo all your hard work.
- Some key areas where your female partner may need a little assistance include helping her to increase the intensity of her exercise, making sure her portions are under control, that she finds methods to deal with stress other than food, positive reinforcement to boost her self-esteem and body image and encouraging her to have a few days each week without food-related treats.
- Some key areas where your male partner may need a little assistance includes helping him access health care when needed, reducing the portion size of his meals, having a few alcohol-free nights each week, learning more about healthy eating, encouraging him to pace himself during exercise and creating some form of incentive or reward for him to change.
- Work on making your partner happy. Be very clear about what's most important to your partner in all aspects of their life. While this book is obviously focused on health, actively helping each other realise your true potential in areas of life such as work, personal development, family, socially and spiritually will only strengthen the bond between you.

Day 28

Include plenty of fibre in your diet

WHAT IS THE IMPACT ON YOUR HEALTH?

Dietary fibre is a component of plant foods that is resistant to digestion and is especially abundant in fruits, vegetables, legumes and grain-based foods. While there are many types of fibre, the three most significant types for your heart health include insoluble fibre, soluble fibre and resistant starch. And they all impact upon your heart health in different ways.

- **Insoluble fibre** contains no kilojoules and provides physical bulk to your diet. It's commonly found in wheat bran, rye and corn, and tends to pass through the intestines undigested, which aids bowel regularity. Foods containing high levels of insoluble fibre can also provide more satisfaction from chewing, giving you a feeling of fullness.

- **Soluble fibre** absorbs water, forming a gel that slows down the digestion of carbohydrate foods, helping to make you feel full. Examples include oat bran, legumes and psyllium husks. This also helps to regulate blood sugar levels and lowers a food's glycemic index. Soluble fibre is like a sponge because it soaks up bile acids that are used to make cholesterol. Fibre itself isn't absorbed, so when it exits the body it takes the bile acids with it. The liver then utilises cholesterol from the blood to produce replacement bile acids, potentially lowering your cholesterol levels.

- **Resistant starch** is a unique type of fibre found in legumes, seeds and nuts, cooked and cooled carbohydrates such as pasta, rice and potato, and intact wholegrain cereals such as oats, rye, wheat, barley, semolina and corn. Because they 'resist' digestion, these foods arrive in larger sized particles in the large intestine. Once there, fermentation produces fatty acids that are absorbed into your bloodstream and these unique fatty acids actually help with weight loss by changing the way the body burns fat as fuel. They are thought to block the body's ability to burn carbohydrates and encourage fat burning sooner. Usually carbohydrates are used first for fuel but when resistant starch is present, stored body fat and recently consumed dietary fat is used earlier as an energy source.

Fibre plays a significant role in weight control. Fibre-rich foods tend to be more filling per kilojoule than other foods, which can help reduce your energy intake. Fibre requires more chewing, which promotes fullness by decreasing your eating speed and increases the release of gastric juices that swell your stomach. Fibre also slows down the rate that glucose is released from foods during digestion, so there is less need for the sugar-and-fat storing hormone insulin. Over the long term this could improve insulin sensitivity and even improve fat oxidation, where your body uses a higher proportion of fat as fuel.

SCIENCE SAYS

More fibre, less heart disease — A 19-year study published in the *Archives of Internal Medicine* found that eating high-fibre foods helps to prevent heart disease. Those who ate the most fibre (around 21 grams per day) had 11 per cent less cardiovascular disease compared to those eating the least fibre (5 grams daily). People eating the most soluble dietary fibre had an even greater improvement in risk reduction.

Fibre helps women's hearts — A six-year study conducted on over 38,000 women that was published in the *Journal of the American College of Cardiology* found that a diet rich in fibre may lower the risk of heart disease in women. Those who ate the most fibre (about 26 grams per day) were less likely to develop heart disease and suffer a heart attack compared with women with a lower fibre intake (about 18 grams a day).

Fibre is a gut-buster — A study reported in the *American Journal of Clinical Nutrition* found that as total fibre intake went up, weight and waist circumference went down. For each 10 grams per day increase in total fibre intake, there was a 0.39 gram per year reduction in weight, and a 0.08 centimetre per year reduction in waist circumference. An additional study reported in the journal *Nutrition* found that subjects who were given an extra 14 grams of fibre per day for 14 weeks lowered their kilojoule intake by 10 per cent and lost around 2 kilograms.

A diversity of fibre is good for the heart — A study reported in *American Journal of Clinical Nutrition* found that a diet that includes diverse sources of fibre may help prevent several major risk factors for heart disease. The study of over 5900 adults aged 35 to 60 found that the higher the participants' fibre intake, the less their risk of being overweight or having elevated blood pressure or cholesterol. The researchers also found that fibre from different sources had somewhat different effects. Fibre from wholegrains, for example, was linked to lower body mass index (BMI), blood pressure and homocysteine (a blood protein connected with heart disease risk). Fruit fibre was associated with lower blood pressure and less abdominal fat, while fibre from vegetables appeared to decrease the risk of high blood pressure and homocysteine. Fibre from nuts and seeds was linked to a lower BMI, a lesser risk of abdominal obesity and healthier blood sugar levels. According to the researchers, these findings stress the importance of getting fibre from a variety of sources.

Psyllium husk lowers cholesterol — According to the US Food and Drug Administration, studies have shown that psyllium husk is effective in lowering total cholesterol and LDL (bad) cholesterol levels. Including 3 to 12 grams of soluble fibre from psyllium seed husk as part of a diet low in saturated fat and cholesterol may reduce the risk of heart disease.

PRACTICAL TIPS ON HOW TO INCLUDE PLENTY OF FIBRE IN YOUR DIET

- As a guide to how much fibre you should have, it's recommended that men eat approximately 35 grams of fibre, and women eat 25 grams each day.
- It can be difficult for people on a low-kilojoule or low-carbohydrate diet to get enough fibre. If you are following one of these dietary regimes pay attention to making sure you get enough fibre.
- When checking labels look for a food that contains at least 4 grams of fibre per 100 grams. Foods with 6 grams or more per serve are considered very good sources of fibre.
- Breakfast is one of the best times of the day to get some fibre in your diet, so try to get your day off to a good start. Some good high-fibre breakfast ideas include baked beans on wholegrain toast or breakfast cereals such as oats, bran flakes and shredded wheat.
- Adding bran to your breakfast cereal is a great way to boost your fibre intake. Some varieties include wheatgerm, wheat bran, oat bran, barley bran, rice bran or psyllium husks.

- A good source of resistant starch is called Hi-Maize, which comes from a special breed of corn. It's used as a food additive in breads, pasta and breakfast cereals without altering the taste, colour or texture of the food. You can also buy it at health food shops and use it instead of flour.
- If you want to sweeten your breakfast cereal use fresh fruit instead of sugar. This will also help boost your nutrient intake.
- Substitute some of the meat in your meals with extra vegetables and/or some of the large varieties of legumes. Legumes are a rich source of fibre.
- The best choices of bread will generally be the varieties that are least processed and that contain seeds and wholegrains. The next best choice is wholemeal, followed by high-fibre white bread and, lastly, plain white bread. Wholegrain bread has twice the fibre content of white bread.
- Choose the brown, wholemeal and wholegrain options for rice, pasta and flour products.
- Try to snack on high-fibre foods like hummus, baked beans, fruit and high-fibre breakfast cereals. Nuts and seeds are also a good source of fibre.
- Where you can, eat the skins of fruit and vegetables such as carrots, potatoes, apples and pears. Removing the skins significantly lowers the fibre and nutrient content of fruits and vegetables.
- Eat some raw vegetables such as carrots, capsicum and celery in salads or as snacks.

- If you struggle to get enough fibre from your diet, fibre supplements may be beneficial.
- If you're making a smoothie add more fibre by including a small amount of oats or psyllium husks. Just let them soak in the milk for a few minutes to soften before blending.

Day 29

Spend less time watching television

WHAT IS THE IMPACT ON YOUR HEALTH?

It may seem surprising but the simple act of watching television is not great for your heart. Television viewing has a strong association with excess body fat, a known risk factor for heart disease. Research has clearly established that as your viewing hours increase so do your chances of being overweight. Television is a sedentary activity and, sadly, many people shift from one seat to another — from the car, to the office and finally to the lounge in front of the television.

It also has an influence over what you eat, where you eat and how much you eat. The following list highlights some of the negative effects that watching television can have on your health.

- It decreases the amount of time you have for planned physical activity.
- It decreases the amount of time you have for planning and preparing healthy meals.
- It is an inactive use of your leisure time.
- It slows down your metabolic rate.
- It can increase your kilojoule intake because of the convenience of nibbling and snacking while viewing.
- People often eat poor quality food in front of the television, which may be related to the influence of junk food advertising.
- Portion sizes may be higher as the distraction of television causes people to overeat.

SCIENCE SAYS

Watch more, weigh more — Several surveys have found that people who watch large amounts of television (3 to 5 hours per day) are fatter than those who watch less. A study conducted at Brigham Young University found that people who watch television 3 or more hours a day are twice as likely to be obese compared to those who watch for less than an hour.

Watch more, eat more — Researchers from the University of Massachusetts found that people who watched television during a meal consumed an average of 1200 more kilojoules than those who didn't. It's believed that watching something on the screen distracts you and keeps your brain from recognising that you're full. The more time spent watching TV, the more kilojoules were eaten.

Metabolism meltdown — According to a study conducted at Memphis State University, your metabolic rate (and kilojoule burning rate) is approximately 14.5 per cent lower when watching television compared to simply lying in bed. It's thought television puts you into a trance-like state that slows down your metabolism. The average person burns off approximately 275 kilojoules per hour, so by not watching television, your body could potentially use an extra 38 kilojoules in that hour, even if you just lie still.

Exercise is no protection — A study reported in the *Journal of the American College of Cardiology* found that watching too much television or playing computer games damages your heart regardless of how much exercise you do. The risk of heart disease and premature death doubled for those spending more than 4 hours a day watching television or playing computer games. The researchers believe that even 2 or more hours of screen time each day may place someone at greater risk of a cardiac event, irrespective of factors such as smoking, hypertension, BMI, and even exercise.

Each hour increases the risk — A study conducted at the Baker IDI Heart and Diabetes Institute in Australia found that every hour spent daily in front of a television increased the chance of death by cardiovascular disease by 18 per cent. This figure was based on a group of people who watched 4 or more hours of television a day and were approximately 80 per cent more likely to develop deadly heart disease than those who watched less than 2 hours.

TV watching narrows the arteries — According to the journal *Thrombosis and Vascular Biology*, children who watch a lot of television tend to have narrow arteries in the back of their eyes, increasing the risk of heart disease, high blood pressure and diabetes later in life. Children who spent at least an hour each day exercising had significantly wider retinal arteries compared to children who were physically active for less than an hour each day.

PRACTICAL TIPS ON HOW TO WATCH LESS TELEVISION

It's ironic that one of the main excuses people give for not exercising is they don't have enough time, yet some people watch several hours of television each day. Television might seem like a great way to unwind but at what price to your health. Imagine what you could achieve by watching less television. It's not about cutting out television, it is about cutting back. Here are a few ideas on just how to do that.

- Limit the amount of time you watch television, videos and DVDs to a set duration, such as 30, 60 or 90 minutes each day.
- Limit the amount of time you spend playing video and computer games.
- Cut back on snacking and eating while watching television. If you do snack while watching television, make sure the food is healthy.

- Only watch the programs you really want to watch.
- Get active while you watch television by doing floor exercises, preparing a healthy meal or using an exercise machine.
- Do something during the ad breaks such as household chores, stretches or moving about.
- Record shows and fast-forward the advertisements to reduce the time you spend in front of the television.
- Have television-free nights on one to two days each week.

Day 30

Lower the GI of your diet

WHAT IS THE IMPACT ON YOUR HEALTH?

The Glycemic Index, or GI, is a ranking system based on how quickly carbohydrate-containing foods release glucose into your bloodstream. Carbohydrates are digested into glucose which is, in turn, absorbed into the bloodstream to supply energy. However, not all carbohydrates release glucose into the bloodstream at the same rate. The faster a food increases your blood sugar levels, the higher will be the insulin response to reduce the escalating blood glucose levels. Foods that release glucose slowly (low GI foods) trigger little if any release of the fat-storing hormone insulin. Low GI foods supply a slow, continuous dose of glucose because they take longer to digest, so they sit in your stomach for longer and make you feel full. The GI classifies carbohydrates more accurately than calling them simple or complex. For example, white rice (formerly thought of as a complex carbohydrate) is absorbed faster than honey (formerly known as a simple carbohydrate).

The benefits to your heart health from eating low GI foods are both direct and secondary. The direct benefit is that people who consume a diet with a lower GI appear to have better cholesterol levels (see 'Science says' below for more details). Keeping your blood sugar levels down is also thought to be heart protective because chronic high levels of blood sugar and insulin cause delicate arteries to become clogged and harden. The secondary benefit to your heart is that a low GI diet can help you lose or maintain a healthy level of body fat. Excess body fat is a known risk factor for heart disease.

SCIENCE SAYS

Lower GI lowers cholesterol — According to the *American Journal of Clinical Nutrition*, there is a strong correlation between HDL (good) cholesterol and the GI of the foods eaten. Subjects with lower GI diets had higher HDL cholesterol levels.

High GI is bad for the heart — A study published in the *American Journal of Clinical Nutrition* found that those who have a diet that contains high GI foods are more prone to developing heart disease. These foods are thought to reduce the levels of good cholesterol in the body while raising triglyceride levels, resulting in narrowing and hardening of the arteries. Subjects with the highest GI diets increase their risk of heart disease by 25 per cent.

High GI and weight gain — Research published in the *Archives of Internal Medicine* found that a low GI diet helps to reduce heart disease risk as well as to lose weight. Women who consumed high GI foods such as white bread and rice had twice as many cases of heart disease as those who consumed a lower than average amount. The researchers believe that high GI foods may prevent the good cholesterol from acting, meaning that the bad cholesterol can do more damage.

Low GI is cardio-protective — A study reported in the *Journal of Nutrition and Metabolism* found that both the quality and the quantity of carbohydrate consumption significantly influenced heart disease risk. People with a low GI and GL (glycemic load) diet (including whole grains, breads, vegetables, legumes, fruits and nuts) had more favourable blood cholesterol and triglyceride (a type of blood fat) concentrations.

Low GI better for fullness — According to the journal *Appetite*, low GI foods delay the return of hunger, decrease subsequent food intake and increase the sensation of fullness compared to high glycemic index foods. The results of several studies suggest that low GI diets also result in significantly more weight or fat loss than high GI diets.

Controlling blood sugar keeps arteries healthy — Findings reported to the American Diabetes Association have shown that diabetics who maintain tight control over their blood sugar can decrease their risk of heart disease. The research was conducted over seven years and found that consistently good blood glucose control resulted in less fatty plaque in the arteries.

PRACTICAL TIPS ON HOW TO LOWER THE GI OF YOUR DIET

- Some supermarket food labels now contain a GI symbol making it easier to choose low GI foods. These foods have been tested using approved methods and will indicate if the food is 'high', 'medium' or 'low' GI.
- Eat plant foods in big chunks. The physical state of a food affects the GI value. Eating whole instead of processed grains and larger chunks of vegetables will slow their absorption. This also helps to minimise food preparation time (for example, you don't need to chop your vegetables up as much) and reduces the food's exposure to oxygen, helping to boost a food's nutrient content.
- Fibre slows down the digestion of carbohydrate foods and helps to lower GI. For example, fruit and vegetables eaten with the skin on (carrots, potatoes, apples and pears) have a lower GI compared to when the skin is removed.
- Combine carbohydrate foods with a source of lean protein. It helps to slow down the digestion of starchy foods from the stomach to the intestine, slowing insulin release and helping to lower their GI. Eating protein with every meal at

the expense of some high GI carbohydrates reduces the need for insulin and allows for greater fat burning.

- Dietary fats slow down the rate that foods leave the stomach, lowering their GI. Diets moderately high in healthy fats can also improve insulin sensitivity, while diets high in saturated and processed fats can induce insulin resistance. The more sensitive your body is to insulin, the less you need and the less fat you will store.

- High acid condiments like lemon juice or vinegar can help to lower the GI of foods. Use lemon juice or balsamic vinegar as a salad dressing or in marinades.

- Focus on improving the quality of your carbohydrates rather than eliminating them as some popular diets encourage you to do. Sure, cut back on carbs, but only the high GI ones such as white bread, white rice and highly processed breakfast cereals. Cutting out all carbs will actually deprive you of foods that taste good, improve bowel health, reduce cholesterol and supply a wide range of vitamins, minerals and antioxidants.

- There are some negative aspects to the GI. Its focus on individual foods rather than whole meals is not always practical (for example, you don't ever really eat pasta on its own) and it also fails to address portion size. Large portions of low GI foods can still trigger a high blood glucose response and therefore be likely to trigger insulin. To address this flaw in the GI, another system of measuring carbohydrates was developed called the glycaemic load. This gives you a figure based on the GI of a food and the serving size, and is a more accurate measure. Practically speaking, the portion size is still important.

- Just as it's important to increase your intake of low GI foods (legumes, oats), it's also important to reduce your intake of high GI foods (cornflakes, white rice).
- The internet is a great reference to find out the GI value of most foods. You can also find pocket books and dietary guides that will list the GI of common foods.

Day 31

Strengthen your muscles

WHAT IS THE IMPACT ON YOUR HEALTH?

Strength training involves adding resistance to your body's natural movements to stimulate muscle strengthening. This resistance can be in the form of your body weight, a hand-held weight such as a dumbbell, pin-loaded weights, hydraulic resistance, elastic bands or water. Strength training (often called weight training or resistance training) has a number of benefits to offer your heart. It has long been used in cardiac rehabilitation programs but it's now recognised for its primary and secondary role as a preventive treatment to reduce the risks of heart disease. It simultaneously engages both the skeletal muscles and the heart and lungs, helping to improve coronary function.

Stronger muscles place fewer demands on the heart, allowing the lungs to process more oxygen with less effort.

The heart can pump more blood with fewer beats (reducing your resting heart rate) and increase the supply of blood flow to your muscles (improving athletic performance). Resistance training helps to lower blood pressure and improve your cholesterol profile (increasing the good, decreasing the bad), while its secondary role is to improve cardiovascular disease risk factors such as body weight, glucose tolerance and insulin sensitivity. It's a great complement to cardiovascular training (running, swimming, cycling) for weight control, giving you more energy, strength and confidence. Strength training also helps to build or maintain lean muscle tissue, which elevates your metabolism and boosts your kilojoule burning rate.

SCIENCE SAYS

Reduced heart rate — According to the *Sports Medicine Journal*, there appears to be a reduction in heart rate from performing resistance training, which is considered beneficial for heart health.

Double bonus — Research published in the *Sports Medicine Journal* has demonstrated favourable changes in both blood fats and cholesterol levels following a strength training intervention.

Combine strength and cardio — A study reported in *Fitness Management Magazine* compared two groups on the same diet for eight weeks, where only one group did 30 minutes of cardiovascular exercise a day, while the other did 15 minutes of cardio combined with 15 minutes of strength training. The cardio and strength training group lost more weight (2 kilograms more), significantly more body fat (3.5 kilograms more) and gained a little more muscle (½ kilogram more).

After-burn bonus — A study reported in the *Journal of Strength and Conditioning Research* showed that subjects who completed an hour-long strength-training workout burn an average of 400 more kilojoules in the 24 hours afterwards than they do when they don't lift weights.

Heart help — The *Journal of the American Medical Association* found that men who lift weights for at least 30 minutes each week had a 23 per cent reduced risk of heart disease compared with those who did not partake in weight training. The researchers claimed that adding weight training to an exercise program is among the most effective strategies to reduce the risk of coronary heart disease in men.

Stroke saviour — According to the journal *Circulation*, stroke survivors who are inactive can develop an intolerance to exercise, resulting in secondary complications such as reduced cardiovascular fitness, muscle wastage, osteoporosis and reduced circulation to the legs. The study authors recommend training using weights or resistance for about 15 repetitions two to three times a week. Typically it's advisable to perform eight to 12 repetitions but for stroke survivors, lighter weights and more repetitions are recommended.

PRACTICAL TIPS TO STARTING A STRENGTH-TRAINING PROGRAM

Don't let the myths about body building hold you back from enjoying the many benefits associated with strength training. The following tips and guidelines are designed to help you get started on a program that will build strength and improve your cardiovascular health. They definitely won't help you build size or bulk.

- Strength training works best as a complement to your cardiovascular exercise, not as a replacement. Aim to do strength-training exercises at least two days a week, making sure you have at least one rest day in between. Your muscles need more time to recover from strength training than they do from moderate intensity aerobic exercise.

- Perform a cardiovascular warm-up for 3 to 5 minutes before doing strength-training exercises. This helps get blood flowing to your muscles and prevents injury.

- Strength-training exercises are described in terms of repetitions and sets. Repetitions are the specific amount of times you perform an exercise, while a set is one group of repetitions of an exercise. For example, doing three sets of 12 push-ups means you would perform 12 push-ups three times.

- Ease yourself gradually into a new strength-training program. Don't perform an exercise to the point where you can't do any more. You should be able to perform at least eight to 15 repetitions of an exercise when starting out;

otherwise, it may be slightly too hard for you. Perform one set of each exercise when starting out and over time build up to two or three.

- Expect to feel some soreness approximately 24 hours after performing strength training for the first three to five times. This is a normal adaptation to a new type of exercise; soon you won't get sore afterwards.
- After the first four to eight weeks, start to push yourself a little harder, increasing the repetitions, sets and/or the amount of weight you lift.
- Always perform strength-training exercises in a controlled manner, keeping your back straight and abdominals contracted. Good technique is vital.
- Perform some light stretching exercises afterwards to prevent soreness. Make sure to target the muscle groups you have trained.
- Each time you perform strength training, aim to do five to 10 different exercises working the legs, chest, arms, back and abdominal muscle groups. At least every four to six weeks try to vary the exercises that you perform for each body part. For example, don't always do just push-ups to strengthen your chest. Include dumbbell and barbell bench press and chest flyes. This prevents overuse injuries and helps develop strength for a wider array of movement patterns.
- Stop immediately if you feel any unusual pain, discomfort or dizziness during strength-training exercises. If you have any doubts, consult a doctor, personal trainer or exercise specialist.

Day 32

Cut back on sugar

WHAT IS THE IMPACT ON YOUR HEALTH?

A major failing of the low-fat approach to losing weight
and improving your health is that it gave people free rein
to overindulge in simple and refined carbohydrates such
as sugar. It's one of the main reasons that low-fat diets are
not that effective unless they address issues like portion
size, sugar and activity levels.

The steadily rising incidence of high blood pressure in
industrialised countries since the 1900s mirrors the global
rise in processed sugar consumption. Manufactured sugar
(which is half fructose and half glucose) is commonly used
in processed and packaged foods. Fructose also occurs
naturally in fruits but the noted increase in fructose
consumption is mainly due to the added sugars in soft
drinks, fruit juice and processed foods. The fructose

in whole fruit also comes loaded with fibre, vitamins, minerals and antioxidants, and is absorbed at a slower rate compared with manufactured fructose, so it is less of a concern. You could say that Mother Nature has packed in a solution (fibre) to the problem (sugar).

Another way that sugar (or more specifically fructose) can impact on your heart health is by increasing uric acid levels in the blood. While the build-up of uric acid is thought to be a primary cause of gout, it is also associated with atherosclerosis (narrowing of the arteries) and high blood pressure. It's also important to know that the body can readily convert an excess of refined carbohydrates (sugars and starches) into saturated fats.

SCIENCE SAYS

Excess sugar equals excess body fat — According to researchers from the University of Minnesota, trends in population-wide weight gain over the past 27 years have paralleled trends in intake of added sugars. While other lifestyle factors should be considered as an explanation for the upward trend of body mass index, the researchers say, efforts should be made to limit added sugar.

Sweet poison — According to the Australian Beverages Council in 2007, Australians drink approximately 110 litres of soft drink each year or around 300 millilitres of regular and diet soft drink per person, per day.

High sugar intake results in hypertension — A study reported in the *Journal of the American Society of Nephrology* found that men who consumed a high sugar diet are more likely to have high blood pressure. Men who consumed 74 grams of fructose a day (around 2.5 cans of soft drink) increased their risk of hypertension by at least 30 per cent. People who consumed even more sugar were more likely to have high blood pressure than people who consumed less. These results occurred independently of other dietary habits such as the intake of salt, carbohydrate and overall kilojoules.

Better to cut back on sugar than carbs — According to the *European Journal of Nutrition*, people hoping to lose weight would be better off cutting out fructose instead of starchy foods such as bread, rice and potatoes. Eating too much fructose causes uric acid levels to spike, which can block the ability of insulin to regulate how the body uses and stores sugar and other nutrients for energy, resulting in obesity and metabolic syndrome.

Sugar increases risk for gout and heart disease — Research reported in the *British Medical Journal* showed that people who consumed two or more sugary soft drinks a day had an 85 per cent higher risk of gout compared with those who drink less than one a month. According to research published in the journal *Arthritis and Rheumatism*, people with gout are at increased risk of having heart health problems.

Milk is better than soft drink — A report in the *American Journal of Clinical Nutrition* found that drinking reduced-fat milk each day may decrease your risk of heart attack. According to the researchers, one explanation for the observed benefit of low-fat dairy products may be that people who drink milk are less likely to drink soft drinks and other highly sugared drinks.

PRACTICAL TIPS TO HELP YOU CUT BACK ON SUGAR

- Avoid adding sugar to foods and drinks such as breakfast cereals, tea and coffee.
- Sugar sweetened soft drinks are high in kilojoules, yet contain minimal, if any, nutrients. Drink water and skim milk instead. Squeeze a little lemon or lime juice in your water if you don't like it plain.
- Fruit juice is extremely high in fructose and is best avoided or watered down. Eat the fruit whole as nature intended and get the additional fibre.
- In addition to eliminating soft drink and fruit juice, cut back on all high sugar beverages like cordial, sports drinks and energy drinks.
- You can choose artificially sweetened drinks to help reduce your sugar intake, although water is a more natural and, in my opinion, a better choice.
- Read food labels and seek out the lower sugar choices. Get to know the alternative names for sugar on food label ingredients lists, such as honey, sucrose, corn syrup, golden syrup and treacle.
- Cut back on packaged and processed foods for which sugar is one of the most common food additives. Instead, try

to eat more whole foods such as fruits, vegetables, lean meats and wholegrains.

- Be wary of foods that contain hidden sugars such as sauces, breakfast cereals, biscuits, spreads and yoghurt.
- Enjoy in moderation high-sugar foods such as cake, chocolate, ice-cream, pastries and desserts and limit them to special occasions.
- Give your tastebuds time to adjust to a diet lower in sugar. It may take several weeks to re-program your palate to less sweetness.
- Fruit is sweet because it's very high in sugar (fructose). Eating too much fruit can still trigger a spike in blood glucose levels and force your body to release insulin — the fat-storing hormone.
- Try to limit your fruit intake to no more than two to three servings a day, especially if you already have high blood pressure or high cholesterol levels.

Day 33

Don't blow your health routine on weekends

WHAT IS THE IMPACT ON YOUR HEALTH?

Weekends can present a serious challenge for people who want to improve their health. It's the ultimate irony. Weekends generally give you more time to exercise and prepare healthy meals, yet people can often overeat, under-exercise and drink alcohol in excess. Other weekend behaviours and habits that can impact upon your heart health include sleeping in (or a change in sleep patterns), hangover-inspired fatty binges, more restaurant meals and fast food, and kilojoule-laden cooked breakfasts. For example, Eggs Benedict contains more kilojoules (2900) than seven chocolate biscuits, and that's without the juice or latte that will often accompany it. Although the impact will vary between individuals, two or three days of overindulgence and under-exercising can make a big difference.

SCIENCE SAYS

High-risk hangover — According to notes in the *British Medical Journal*, weekend binge drinking may be linked to heart attacks. It's thought that alcohol, particularly when consumed in a binge, acts as a trigger for a heart attack. There was almost a two-fold increase in the risk of having a heart attack during a severe hangover. Binge drinking causes dehydration and may actually promote clotting after the heavy drinking stops. It also changes heart rhythms, increases blood pressure and may damage the lining of blood vessels and the heart muscle, all placing extra pressure on the heart.

Weekend weight gain — A study published in the journal *Obesity* examined people's diet and activity patterns, and weighed them daily over several years. The researchers found that subjects consistently gained weight on weekend days (Friday, Saturday and Sunday) but not on weekdays (Monday to Thursday). This was found to be from a higher energy intake and lower levels of physical activity on weekends. The average weekend weight gain was 0.077 kilograms, which may seem small; however, if this rate continued throughout the year it would result in an annual weight gain of 4 kilograms. It was also reported that people whose diets were less consistent between weekdays and weekends were more likely to gain weight during the subsequent year.

Weekend kilojoule binge — Research reported in the journal *Obesity* found the effects of weekend days on kilojoule intake was substantial. It was found that taking an average of all age groups, the subjects of the study consumed an extra 1033 kilojoules on weekends compared with weekdays. This could result in an annual weight gain of 1.5 kilograms. The researchers noted that adults aged 19 to 50 should be particularly aware of their health on weekends because they consumed an extra 1449 kilojoules on weekends. The increased kilojoule consumption was primarily from extra fat and alcohol consumption.

Weekends are a heart danger zone for middle-aged men — A French study published in the journal *Heart* found that middle-aged men are more likely to die from a heart attack on Saturday or Sunday than during the work week. It was found that 25- to 54-year-old men had a 20 per cent greater risk of dying from a heart attack on the weekend than mid-week.

Eat breakfast at home — *The American Journal of Epidemiology* reported that regularly eating breakfast away from home (a common weekend pastime) was associated with excess body fat, significantly increasing the chances of being overweight. Breakfast eaten away from home was much higher in kilojoules and fat, containing more saturated fat and less fibre compared with breakfasts eaten at home.

Learn from the losers — A study published in the *American Journal of Clinical Nutrition* tracked more than

4000 people who had lost over 12 kilograms and kept it off for more than 12 months. One of the common habits was that they maintained a consistent eating pattern, varying it very little on weekends or holidays. Those who were less strict about their regimen on weekends and holidays tended to put weight back on.

Be consistent — A study reported in the journal *Obesity* found that overindulging at weekends makes it hard to maintain lost weight. They found people who eat consistently seven days a week are more likely to keep off weight than those who watched what they ate only on weekdays.

PRACTICAL TIPS ON HOW TO AVOID BLOWING YOUR HEALTH ROUTINE ON WEEKENDS

- Take advantage of the extra time you have by getting outside and doing a long workout. You can also try activities that may be harder to participate in before or after work. Physical activity actually gives you more energy to cope with the weekly grind.
- Combine social time involving family and friends with physical activity. There are plenty of ways you can have fun and get active such as taking a ball or frisbee on a picnic, swimming at the beach or going for a family bush walk.
- Use the weekends to get organised with your food by planning your meals for the week and making some healthy big batch meals to freeze. It also helps to plan ahead for parties and social events by eating a healthy meal beforehand or taking some healthy food with you.

- Try to keep your eating routine as normal and consistent as possible by always watching your intake of fat, fast food and alcohol, especially on weekends. Balance out any indulgences by consuming moderate portions, having smaller portions of other foods before and afterwards, and performing extra exercise.
- If you have a hot breakfast, choose healthier ingredients like poached eggs, egg white omelets, baked beans, grilled tomatoes, steamed spinach and wholegrain toast without butter. Try to limit your intake of bacon, fried eggs, hash browns, Hollandaise sauce and breakfast sausages.
- If you only tend to exercise on weekends, have a look at your schedule and see if you can squeeze in one to two mid-week workouts. Even if it's just 20 minutes during your lunch break or a quick workout after work, this can give your body a much stronger foundation for activity.
- Weekend warriors (people who only exercise on weekends) may be more prone to injuries. To reduce your risk and increase the enjoyment of your chosen activity, make sure you warm up, take short rests during your workout when needed, progress gradually and cool down afterwards.
- Re-think the way you treat yourself. If you feel like you deserve an indulgence or treat after a long week, try to use rewards that are not centred around food or alcohol. This might include renting a DVD, buying a book or magazine or having a bath. Try to avoid rewards that undo all your work during the week.

Day 34

Be wise about your hot drinks

WHAT IS THE IMPACT ON YOUR HEALTH?

Looking at how hot drinks like tea and coffee can impact on your health is complicated. There are a number of variables, including the caffeine and antioxidant content in your drink of choice, what you have to accompany it, and the behaviours associated with drinking tea and coffee. Let's look at these issues separately.

Caffeine — The caffeine in tea and coffee makes it the most widely consumed stimulant in the world. On one hand, consuming a caffeinated drink such as black coffee (it must have no sugar or milk to be effective) before exercise can actually boost fat-burning. But an excessive intake of caffeine can cause insomnia, stomach complaints, anxiety and irritability in some people. Over the long term there is some evidence to suggest that drinking a lot of caffeinated beverages can impact negatively on your cholesterol levels and bone density.

Antioxidants — Hot drinks are one of the best sources of antioxidants in a typical diet. While green tea and black tea come from the same plant, green tea is minimally processed, resulting in less oxidation and a much richer concentration of nutrients and antioxidants. Green tea contains EGCG (epigallocatechin-3-gallate), an antioxidant compound that is thought to lower your cholesterol and blood pressure levels. Coffee is also rich in antioxidants but the higher caffeine content may negate some benefits. There is also some research to suggest that milk, when added to tea or coffee, neutralises the benefits of antioxidants (see 'Science says' below for more details).

Accompaniments — When you add sugar, milk and even cream to your cup of tea or coffee, the kilojoule and fat content escalates dramatically. The foods that often accompany tea and coffee are also high in kilojoules and fat, such as biscuits, doughnuts, cakes, pastries and desserts. Many of these foods contain trans fats, the worst kind of dietary fat for your heart.

Associated behaviours — Coffee and, to a lesser extent, tea, are associated with behaviours known to tax the heart, including sleeplessness and stress. There is some research to suggest that people who drink coffee also tend to have more fat in their diet.

Black tea blocks fat — A study reported in the journal *Nutrition* has shown that extracts from tea leaves may help with weight loss. According to the researchers, tea contains high levels of polyphenols (a type of antioxidant), which block fat absorption and reduce cholesterol levels. However, the proteins in cow's milk cancel out these health benefits. According to the researchers, this phenomenon might explain why people in Britain do not appear to benefit from the healthy effects of tea despite being among the world's biggest consumers of the beverage.

Black tea is good for the blood — A study reported in the *European Journal of Clinical Nutrition* found that drinking tea without milk (black, oolong or green) may lower the risk of heart disease by preventing the blood from forming clots. Sticky blood can more easily form clots, which can block the flow of blood through the body and lead to a heart attack.

Have a black coffee before exercise — A study reported in the *Journal of Medicine and Science in Sport* found that consuming caffeine (in the form of black coffee) an hour before exercise made a significant difference to fat use. The caffeine-consuming athletes used an amazing 107 per cent more fat as fuel compared to those on a placebo.

Have black tea after a fatty meal — According to the American Society for Clinical Nutrition, the harmful effects of a fatty meal may be reduced by following it up with a cup of black tea. Subjects who ate a meal containing approximately 80 per cent fat and then drank black tea afterwards had signs of improved blood flow compared to those who only drank water afterwards. The researchers suggested that the antioxidants in black tea may help to prevent the temporary stiffening and constriction of blood vessels associated with elevated blood fat levels which occur after a high-fat meal.

Black tea is good for heart attack survivors — Research published in *Circulation*, the journal of the American Heart Association, found that heart attack sufferers who drank at least 14 cups of black tea each week survived longer than those who didn't drink tea. According to the researchers, black tea helps the blood vessels' ability to relax, especially in individuals with existing heart disease. They also cited other research which found the flavanoids present in tea prevent LDL (bad) cholesterol from oxidising and sticking to the artery walls, and may prevent blood clots from forming.

Green tea has small fat loss benefits — A study reported in the *American Journal of Clinical Nutrition* found that a green tea extract consumed three times a day increased metabolic rate by approximately 4 per cent over 24 hours. Fat oxidation (the proportion of fat used as fuel) was also higher for people taking the green tea extract (41.5 per cent) compared to those on a placebo (31.6 per cent).

Heavy coffee drinking weighs heavily on the heart —
A study reported in the *American Journal of Epidemiology*
found that drinking six cups of coffee a day was associated
with an increase in total cholesterol, LDL (bad) cholesterol
and triglycerides, but not HDL (good) cholesterol levels. It
was thought that coffee oils were the main reason behind
the cholesterol-raising effect because filtered coffee
had less impact on raising cholesterol levels. Still, it is
important to note that there are some conflicting studies
on the impact of coffee on the heart and more conclusive
research is needed.

Coffee may damage blood vessels — A report presented
to the European Society of Cardiology showed that drinking
coffee may cause damage to your blood vessels. Test
subjects who drank 250 milligrams of caffeine (equivalent
to two or three cups of coffee) experienced a loss of aortic
elasticity and raised blood pressure levels. The aorta is the
main artery supplying blood to the body.

PRACTICAL TIPS ON HOW TO BE WISE ABOUT YOUR HOT DRINKS

The following tips are designed to maximise the heart
health benefits of hot drinks and minimise any negative
health effects.

- Cut out or at least cut back on the amount of sugar you
  have in your tea or coffee. After a month or two you won't
  even miss it.

- To help reduce your kilojoule intake and boost the antioxidant content of your diet try to have no milk with your tea or coffee. The proteins in milk may neutralise the effectiveness of antioxidant compounds. If you can't survive without milk, use skim to minimise your saturated fat intake. As with reducing your intake of sugar, your tastebuds may take a month or two to adapt.
- Don't accompany your hot drinks with foods such as biscuits, pastry, cake, doughnuts or muffins that can outweigh any potential benefits.
- If you are eating foods with your hot drinks be careful of your portion size. Caffeine is a known stimulant and can increase your appetite.
- A good choice of hot drinks is green tea, which is available as loose leaf and in tea bags. Oolong tea is processed less than black tea but more than green tea. To maximise the antioxidant content of tea, add water that is allowed to stand for a few minutes after boiling. This is because antioxidants are damaged by heat.
- Try not to use tea and coffee as a form of stress relief. Day 36 talks of other ways to relax to relieve stress.
- To minimise the impact on your sleep quality and quantity avoid having tea and coffee within a few hours of bedtime.
- While coffee and tea are high in antioxidants they cannot replace fruits and vegetables, which supply fibre, important vitamins and minerals, plus a wider diversity of antioxidants.
- If you have a cappuccino or latte, choose the skinny option. The amount of milk you consume will vary depending on

whether your coffee is a small, medium or large, but you could be consuming between one and two cups of milk. Every cup of full cream milk has 9.5 grams of fat and 300 kilojoules above and beyond what you'd get in a cup of skim milk.

- The health benefits from tea and coffee come from drinking it black and in moderation. Try to limit your intake to no more than two cups of coffee or three cups of tea a day.

Day 35

Manage your workplace health, especially if you are stressed or desk-bound

WHAT IS THE IMPACT ON YOUR HEALTH?

It's not uncommon to spend a third of your adult life at work, so your workplace environment will have a significant impact on your overall health. Changes in our work culture, including a dramatic reduction in physically active jobs, has led to a large increase in the number of people who are unhealthy because of inactivity and excess weight. Too much sitting is not good for your body or your heart. The age of information has also brought about rapid change in work practices: a quick voicemail, email, fax, or mobile phone call or text can shif the focus of your effort several times a day. Workplace stress has become a modern epidemic and it has many causes, although generally it involves a combination of high demands with a low level of control. Increasing pressures from deadlines, traffic to and from work, computers, long working hours and possible conflicts with co-workers are just a few of the issues many people have to face.

SCIENCE SAYS

Clot risk for desk jockeys — According to the *European Respiratory Journal*, sitting in front of the computer for hours on end could increase the risk of blood clots. The researchers compared it to the increased risk of blood clots associated with long-distance air travel. They suggested people who sit for prolonged periods would benefit from frequent leg and foot exercises as well as regular mobilisation breaks such as a short walk or stretch.

Workplace stress clusters — Research reported in the *British Medical Journal* found that prolonged exposure to workplace stress can contribute to the development of a cluster of health problems, including heart disease. Men with chronic work stress had nearly double the odds of developing metabolic syndrome (a precursor to heart disease) compared to those with no exposure to work stress. You are thought to suffer from metabolic syndrome (also known as syndrome X) if you have three or more of the following symptoms: high blood pressure, abdominal obesity, low HDL (good) cholesterol, high triglycerides and elevated fasting blood glucose levels.

Job stress and blood pressure — A study published in the *American Journal of Epidemiology* found that workers who spend years in a high-stress job had a large increase in blood pressure both when they were on the job and at home. Stressed out men had an increase of 6 to 8 points in systolic blood pressure (the upper number in the blood pressure reading) compared to workers in low-stress jobs.

Supportive environment important — According to the *American Journal of Public Health*, people with low levels of support from their supervisors and/or co-workers are at a high risk of increased blood pressure. The study was conducted on over 6500 men and women, and involved an initial questionnaire with a 7.5-year follow-up. Also of interest was the fact that men with the most job strain were 33 per cent more likely to experience an increase in blood pressure.

Noise is a major health hazard for men — Findings reported in the *Heart Journal* showed that chronic noise at work can increase stress levels, which may set off changes in the body that can trigger a heart attack. Although women were not affected by noise in the workplace, it increased the risk of a heart attack by a third in men.

Long work hours are like hard labour to your heart — A study reported in the *Annals of Internal Medicine* journal which followed more than 7000 workers over 11 years found that regularly working long hours can significantly raise the risk of heart disease. The researchers found that working more than 11 hours a day increased the risk of heart disease by 67 per cent, compared with working 7 to 8 hours a day. It's uncertain if the long working hours contribute to the increased risk of heart disease themselves or whether they are a trigger for other unhealthy behaviours such as a poor diet, inactivity and stress.

PRACTICAL TIPS ON HOW TO MANAGE YOUR WORKPLACE HEALTH

- **Manage your time** — Set realistic goals and deadlines and plan work projects in advance. Make lists and priorities and schedule all the important aspects of your life, including work and health, relationships and family.
- **Accumulate your exercise** — Use short bouts of exercise to accumulate activity over the day and incorporate more movement into your lifestyle. For example, a 10-minute walk before work, a 10-minute walk to get a sandwich at lunch, and a 10-minute walk from the bus on the way home.
- **Get active in your lunch break** — This is ideal if you are an early starter or often feel too tired when you get home at night. You don't have to sweat for your heart to benefit. Alternatively, take a change of clothes and go a little harder.
- **Don't skip breakfast** — When you're running late or not hungry first thing in the morning it can be easy to skip breakfast. Yet this can leave you tired and hungry by mid-morning, making it more likely that you'll snack on junk food later in the day. Be prepared and have foods you can eat in

the car, bus or train such as fruit, breakfast bars, breakfast drinks or a low-fat bran muffin.

- **Be organised with your workplace lunch** — Plan ahead of time and make a sandwich, salad or soup the night before. Go for lunches that include wholegrains, lean meats and vegetables.
- **Thirsty work** — Drink plenty of water at work, especially if your office is air-conditioned. Be especially careful to avoid soft drink vending machines and full-fat milk drinks.
- **Snack well** — Munch on fresh and canned fruit between meals. Take fruits to work that are easy to store and eat, like an apple, pear, mandarin or banana. Other snack ideas include nuts and unsweetened low-fat natural yoghurt.
- **Back care** — Most people will experience back pain at some stage of their life and occupational back pain accounts for a quarter of all compensated injuries. Back pain can be debilitating and may put a halt to your activity levels (which are vital for heart health). With the majority of people working in a seated position it is important that you have a workstation that is ergonomically designed to suit you and your needs.
- **Take mini breaks** — Stretching and moving is a great way to counteract the small repetitive movements that are commonplace in most workplaces. Take 30 seconds every hour to get away from your computer and desk and recharge your body. Stretching and exercise helps to stimulate blood flow and boost your energy levels while also helping to prevent tension, fatigue and stiffness.

- **Take regular holidays** — Try not to accrue your leave. Regular holidays help you avoid exhaustion and burnout. They also help you reconnect with your friends and family, and give you renewed job satisfaction when you return in a refreshed state.

- **Be aware of occupational health and safety practices** — Don't let a workplace injury interfere with your quality or quantity of life. Be aware of safe workplace practices. For example, wear ear protection if you experience chronic noise at work. Chronic exposure to loud noise is actually linked to heart disease.

- **A warning to workaholics** — If you work long hours (more than 8 hours a day), pay careful attention to eating well, being physically active, managing stress and keeping your blood pressure, cholesterol and blood sugar levels within healthy limits.

Day 36

Make time for relaxation

WHAT IS THE IMPACT ON YOUR HEALTH?

Relaxation is a break from your work or activities involving rest or pleasant recreation (although it isn't sleep). It allows your body to release tension and leads to physical and emotional changes that are opposite to the stress response. It can strengthen your physical and emotional reserves to help cope with future stress. Relaxation slows your heart rate and reduces blood pressure, making life easier on your heart. By pushing the pause button and relaxing for even just a few moments, you can re-boot your energy levels and rejuvenate your body. However, just as stress affects individuals differently, what is relaxing for some is not for others. It's important to choose a relaxation technique that is suitable for you and most likely to relieve the type of stress (physical or emotional) you often experience.

SCIENCE SAYS

Relaxation boosts weight loss — A study reported in the journal *Preventive Medicine* found that women who meditated and did yoga lost an average of 2.5 kilograms over two years compared to those who focused purely on exercise and nutrition. The researchers believed that reducing stress stops cravings for fatty foods and sweets. By learning and practising relaxation techniques as part of a wider lifestyle change program, the study participants had effective tools to manage stress and emotions without resorting to unhealthy eating.

Yoga cuts stress hormones — Medical research has discovered a strong connection between yoga and stress relief. A study conducted at the Thomas Jefferson University in the United States found that after a single 50-minute session of yoga, levels of the stress hormone cortisol dropped, even in people who were trying yoga for the first time.

Meditation calms the mind and the heart — A study conducted by the *American Journal of Cardiology* has found that meditation may not only reduce stress, but also may help adults with high blood pressure to live longer. Participants were followed for approximately eight years on average, and the group who practised meditation not only had lower blood pressure than those in a control group but were also 30 per cent less likely to die from cardiovascular disease.

Tai chi relieves anxiety — A study reported in the *Archives of Internal Medicine* reviewed the health benefits of tai chi and found it was effective in providing relief from stress and anxiety. While considered a form of exercise, its movements are slow, fluid, calm and controlled, concentrating on deep breathing, balance, form and mental imagery.

PRACTICAL TIPS ON HOW TO RELAX MORE

- Take a few minutes each day to escape all the noise. Turn off the phone and the television and feel yourself unwind by enjoying a brief period of quiet time.
- Immerse yourself in a warm bath or spa to help loosen tense muscles and feel relaxed. Add scented oils or bath salts to further set the mood. The feeling of cleanliness after washing is also refreshing.
- Deep breathing is a quick, easy, cheap and natural way to help counter the effects of stress. Increasing your oxygen intake through conscious, deeper breathing can help you relax, increasing your energy levels. Take a slow, deep breath in through your nose for a count of three, then out through your mouth for a count of four, and repeat 10 times.
- Go for a light walk to get away from a stressful environment. It doesn't have to be an exercise walk, more like a short escape. Short bursts of activity such as walking or stretching help to boost your circulation and clear your mind.

- Include mind/body exercise such as yoga, tai chi and pilates in your training schedule. These activities engage your mind and help you to relax, getting you to focus on posture, form, breathing and the abdominal core. The slow, controlled movements are generally low impact.
- Listening to slow, soothing music can also help you unwind and calm your mood. Find a collection of songs that calm you and call on them when you need time out.
- Massage is a form of physical relaxation that helps to improve circulation and relax tired muscles. Massage therapy also promotes a unique feeling of wellbeing that helps to release tension and prevents stress.
- Meditation is a very effective method of relaxation and stress reduction. It lets you take a conscious break from thoughts and distraction, slowing down your heart rate and breathing rate and relaxing your muscles. The intention is to enter a state of 'restful alertness', in which the body is awake but the mind is not engaged in conscious thought.
- You can purchase books, CDs and mp3 tracks to help you relax. These might include recordings of white noise, whale sounds, the sounds of the ocean or rainforest, or specific relaxation techniques designed to help you unwind.
- Stretching not only lengthens your muscles and tendons, it can also help you to relax, calm the mind and relieve some of the day's stressors. It helps to counter muscle tension from work, stress and exercise by extending the range of motion of your muscles and joints, improving circulation and promoting better posture. By focusing your mind on the

body part you're stretching, you can also take your mind off other stressful thoughts. You can also combine stretching with deep breathing to maximise the stress-relieving effect.

- Don't stockpile your annual leave when you could be forgetting all your troubles somewhere peaceful. Take your holidays and give your body regular breaks to help rest, relax, repair and recuperate. Even a day off or a long weekend can clear your mind and renew your energy levels.

Day 37

Change the way you eat chocolate

WHAT IS THE IMPACT ON YOUR HEALTH?

Chocolate is often looked upon as an indulgent treat that contributes to weight gain. Yet the impact that chocolate has on your heart health can be either positive or negative depending on the type and quantity you eat. All chocolate is made from the bitter cacao bean, which undergoes a number of processes (including fermentation, drying, roasting and grinding) to form the key ingredients of chocolate — cocoa butter and cocoa. Cocoa contains fibre and polyphenol compounds that have antioxidant and possible anti-inflammatory properties and may boost heart health in a similar way to tea and red wine. But to make chocolate, other ingredients are added such as sugar and dairy products that can add significant amounts of kilojoules and fat. The quality, processing and ratio of ingredients in chocolate will determine what impact it has on your health. As a general rule, the darker the chocolate, the greater the health benefits. Dark chocolate contains 70 per cent or more cocoa and it is the only type of chocolate that could be described as healthy. White chocolate contains cocoa butter but little or no actual cocoa, while milk chocolate is too high in sugar and dairy fats and too low in cocoa to have a positive influence on heart health.

SCIENCE SAYS

Chocolate has antioxidant properties — According to a study published in the *American Journal of Clinical Nutrition*, compounds found in chocolate called catechins may help protect against heart disease. Catechins are part of a group of plant compounds called flavonoids, an antioxidant linked to a lower risk of a number of diseases and cancers. Elderly men who consumed the most catechins (also found in green tea and fruit) were 51 per cent less likely to die of heart disease over a 10-year period. Additional research reported in the *Chemistry Central Journal* found that cocoa powder and dark chocolate actually had a greater antioxidant capacity than fruit juice.

Dark chocolate is a bright spot for heart health — A study published in *Heart* magazine found that a few squares of dark chocolate every day might cut the risk of serious heart disease by helping to stave off the hardening of arteries. Two groups of smokers ate 40 grams of either dark or white chocolate. After two hours, tests revealed that the dark chocolate (74 per cent cocoa) significantly improved the smoothness of arterial flow, while white chocolate (4 per cent cocoa) had no effect.

Just a sniff, thanks — According to the journal *Regulatory Peptides*, even the smell of dark chocolate can have an appetite-suppressing effect. The study on a group of young women found that eating 30 grams of dark chocolate (85 per cent cocoa) reduced hunger. But more surprising was the fact that women who only smelt the chocolate still experienced a reduction in appetite, which can help reduce the risk of overeating. Women who sniffed the dark chocolate had lower levels of the appetite-stimulating hormone ghrelin, and the researchers believe that it may be possible, by using certain food odours, to 'trick' the brain into believing it had been fed.

Chocolate improves blood vessel function — A study published in the *American Journal of Clinical Nutrition*, showed that eating dark chocolate could significantly improve (blood vessel) function. During the six-week trial subjects were given either 227 grams of cocoa without sugar, 227 grams of cocoa with sugar, or a placebo each day. A measure of blood flow found the cocoa without sugar brought about improvements by 2.4 per cent, and the cocoa with sugar improved blood flow by 1.5 per cent. There was a minimal difference in the placebo group.

According to the researchers, this demonstrates one way that the flavonoids in dark chocolate provide cardiovascular benefits.

PRACTICAL TIPS ON CHANGING THE WAY YOU EAT CHOCOLATE

- If you are going to eat chocolate to benefit your heart make sure it's dark chocolate that contains at least 70 per cent cocoa.
- Cut back on or minimise your intake of white chocolate and dairy milk chocolate. These foods have a detrimental effect on heart health.
- Dark chocolate is still a high-kilojoule, high-fat food, so limit your portion size. Some studies have shown there are benefits from eating as little as 30 grams a day. If you do eat larger portions of chocolate, cut out other sweets or snacks or perform extra exercise to balance out the extra kilojoule intake.
- Skip the additives that often come with chocolate such as caramel, nougat or cream fillings, which just add extra sugar and fat. If you like something extra with your dark chocolate, eat it with some raw, unsalted nuts.
- Avoid washing your chocolate down with a glass of cow's milk. Just as the milk in tea or coffee is thought to negate any antioxidant effects, the same applies to chocolate. A heart healthy way to get your hot chocolate fix is by using cocoa powder and almond, oat, soy or rice milk. Just keep the sugar content to a minimum.

Day 38

Get a dog

WHAT IS THE IMPACT ON YOUR HEALTH?

Pets have a very positive impact on many aspects of our health with research showing that pet owners experience some unique heart health benefits. Interaction with domesticated animals is thought to decrease blood pressure and heart rate, and also offer psychological and emotional benefits. But the real advantage of dog ownership over other domesticated pets is that they make excellent workout partners, serving as a ready source of motivation to keep you active on a regular basis. Some of the reasons that dogs make such good exercise companions include:

- They like to be walked every day.
- They are ready to go when you are.
- They never have an excuse not to exercise.

- They provide added safety during your exercise.
- They make you feel guilty if they don't get walked.
- They can behave badly if they don't get walked.
- They don't slow down for hills.
- They can vary their speed to suit you.
- You will probably wear out before they do.

The benefits of walking or running with your dog include improved stamina, weight management by burning off kilojoules and the opportunity to enjoy the great outdoors. These benefits will also extend to your four-legged friend.

SCIENCE SAYS

Pets help after heart attack — Research published in the *American Journal of Cardiology* has found that after a heart attack pet owners have healthier hearts than heart attack patients who don't have a dog or cat. Owning a pet, particularly a dog, was associated with improved measures of heart rate variability, which is an indicator of the heart's ability to handle stress. Pet ownership is also known to increase the 12-month survival rate after people have been hospitalised for heart problems.

Lower cholesterol and triglycerides — According to the *Medical Journal of Australia*, people with pets have been found to have lower cholesterol and triglyceride levels when compared to people who did not have pets, even when accounting for weight, diet and smoking habits.

Pet ownership lowers blood pressure — According to the journal *Hypertension*, pet owners with long-term animal exposure had lower measures of blood pressure and heart rate compared to people who were not pet owners.

Dogs boost weight loss — A study reported in the journal *Obesity* compared a group of overweight people on a combined owner/dog program of diet and exercise with people who also dieted and exercised but who acted alone. For 12 months both groups followed a kilojoule-controlled diet and 20- to 30-minute walks on most days of the week. While both groups lost a similar amount of weight, participants who trained with their dogs were more effective at maintaining participation in physical activity. According to the researchers, the dog owners were more confident and motivated to follow the diet and exercise program and succeed at weight loss, both in the short and the long run. Out of interest, the dogs also lost around 15 per cent of their body weight, showing the benefits extend to both man and beast alike.

PRACTICAL TIPS ON MAXIMISING THE HEALTH BENEFITS OF DOG OWNERSHIP

- The breed and size of your dog will determine how fast and, generally, how effective your shared exercise sessions are. Medium to large dogs such as labradors or beagles will allow you to walk faster and even run, while smaller dogs such as terriers or dachshunds still enjoy a short walk and can add some fun to your exercise routine.
- If you intend to do a lot of running it may be best to look towards a breed of sporting dog, such as a retriever.

- If you have been exercising for several months and your fitness is at a good level, incorporate some interval training into your combined workouts. Find a suitable open space and perform several faster runs, followed by slow walking to catch your breath. It's a great way to up the intensity of your workouts and most dogs will enjoy it too.
- If your dog constantly stops to sniff things or play around, go to puppy or dog training school. A rhythmic and continuous walk will offer you both more health benefits. If your dog is too old to learn new tricks add an extra walk or run afterwards (by yourself) to get the maximum health benefits.
- A well-trained dog should allow you to maintain a good steady pace at a level where you can hear your breath. This 'breath test' is a good indicator that you are exercising at the right intensity.
- Remember to keep both of you well hydrated before, during and after your workout, especially on hot days. It's also best for both of you to exercise on an empty stomach (unless you are diabetic). You'll potentially burn more fat while your dog will be less likely to experience bloating.
- Try not to rely on exercise with your dog as your only source of physical activity for weight control. Use it as a complement to other, more intense activities.
- Don't forget to take a lead and a plastic bag, and be aware of providing a comfortable space between your dog and other walkers.

Day 39

Choose healthy snack foods in healthy portions

WHAT IS THE IMPACT ON YOUR HEALTH?

The concept of a snack as a 'between meal' filler has changed in modern times as snacking has evolved into a fourth meal of the day. There are estimates that snacks can make up 20 to 30 per cent of people's kilojoule intakes with snack foods also sneaking their way into meal times as accompaniments or replacements.

The impact snacking can have on your heart health can vary dramatically depending on a number of variables, such as the quality of the snack, the portion size of the snack and the portion size of your other meals. In terms of the quality of the snack there is a big difference between snacking on fruit compared to snacking on potato crisps. A lot of snack foods are high in sugar, fat and salt — the three danger nutrients when it comes to heart health. However, healthy snacks that are moderate to low in kilojoules and high in nutrients can help to manage your weight by controlling hunger levels and preventing bingeing between meals.

Snacking may help to prevent cravings and boost your energy levels, but it will only work to improve your health if your overall kilojoule intake does not increase. If the portion size of the snack itself is too large or if the portion size of your other meals is not reduced to compensate for snacking, you will still end up consuming too many kilojoules. This can result in weight gain, a significant risk for heart disease.

SCIENCE SAYS

Snack more, eat more — A study published in the *Journal of the American Dietetic Association* found that the more often a person eats in a day, the more kilojoules they are likely to consume. This emphasises the importance of watching the portion sizes of your main meals if you snack regularly.

Too many snack choices are dangerous — A study reported in *Psychological Bulletin* found that when faced with multiple snacking options people may eat beyond the point of hunger in order to get a taste of all that is before them. Put practically, a person who has a kitchen full of various goodies might chow down on more kilojoules than a person who stocks only one snack choice.

Snacking not needed for weight loss — A study from the University of Newcastle had two groups of people eat the same foods and the same amount of kilojoules. However, one group divided their kilojoule intake into six portions while the other group ate three square meals. The research found there was no significant difference in the amount of weight either group lost. So whether you snack or not, the key is to keep your total kilojoule intake under control.

An apple a day — According to the *American Journal of Clinical Nutrition*, there may be some truth to the theory that an apple a day keeps the doctor away. They found men who ate the most catechins (a compound found in apples), were 51 per cent less likely to die of heart disease over 10 years, compared with men who consumed the least. Catechins are also found in other fruits, red wine and tea.

PRACTICAL TIPS ON CHANGING THE WAY YOU SNACK

- Don't feel compelled to snack because you think it will help you lose weight. You don't actually need to snack at all and three square meals work fine for some people. For others, snacking is a way of life due to the hunger they experience between meals. Identify what times of day you are most likely to snack and plan to have healthy snack foods available.

- Healthy snacks work best when they are coordinated with the portion size of your main meals. If you snack regularly it's best to eat less at breakfast, lunch or dinner.

- It's also important to adjust your snacking depending on your activity levels. Try to snack less and reduce your kilojoule intake on the days you don't exercise. In addition it's important to not go overboard and eat too much on the days when you are active. Exercise can trigger a hunger sensation that is greater than your actual kilojoule needs, so drink plenty of water and eat slowly when you do snack.
- Snack on exercise instead of food. Just as you might look towards a small snack of food to give you an energy boost or improve your mood, why not use exercise to do the same? Short bites of activity can distract you when you're tempted to indulge, helping to keep hunger pangs at bay.
- Clear your home of any unhealthy snacks and stock up with healthy choices. If high-salt, high-fat and high-sugar snacks are harder to come by you won't be so tempted to have them. Some snack foods to avoid include banana bread, fruit juice, soft drink, potato crisps, milk chocolate bars, sweet biscuits, pastries and choc chip muesli bars.
- Plan ahead by taking a healthy snack with you to work, school or the park. That way you won't be tempted to snack on junk. You can also take your own healthy snack foods to parties and social gatherings so there is at least one healthy choice available.
- Popcorn makes for a great snack but only if it's air-popped. Use spices such as cumin, cayenne pepper, garlic salt or chicken salt to add flavour without oil or butter. Oil-popped or movie-theatre popcorn usually contains over three times the kilojoule content of air-popped.

- Fresh fruit, canned fruit and fruit salad are all an OK snack choice but they are all reasonably high in sugar, so don't go overboard with your portions.
- Nuts are a good snack but watch your portion size. Try to keep it to a small handful, using nuts that haven't been roasted or salted such as cashews, almonds or walnuts. Buy them in bulk and place individual servings in small zip-lock bags to take with you.
- Try to vary the type of foods you snack on, which makes your food more enjoyable and helps you get a wider range of nutrients from your diet. Ideally, snacks should be no more than 400 to 600 kilojoules. Some healthy snack ideas include low-salt vegetable-based soups, vegetable sticks (carrot, celery, red capsicum) with salsa, baked beans on wholegrain toast, cracker bread with cottage cheese and avocado, low-fat natural yoghurt with chopped fruit and high-fibre breakfast cereal with skim milk.
- Avoid drinking sugary drinks between meals if you're feeling a little hungry. Have a glass of water instead.
- Be wary of low-fat snacks. A number of processed low-fat or reduced-fat foods such as biscuits, cakes, muffins, yoghurts and ice-cream still have significant amounts of sugar and kilojoules. Just because something is 97 per cent fat-free doesn't necessarily mean it will boost your heart health.

Day 40

Indulge in these extras to your heart's content

GET ENOUGH MAGNESIUM IN YOUR DIET

Magnesium is important for cellular energy production and has muscle-tension relieving properties. Signs of low magnesium levels can include fatigue, irritability, muscle cramps and a predisposition to stress. A study on 7000 adults reported in the *American Journal of Cardiology* found that a greater intake of magnesium appears to reduce the risk of heart disease. Over 15 years, those with the lowest daily magnesium intake (186 milligrams or less) had nearly double the rate of heart disease compared to those with the highest daily magnesium intake (340 milligrams or more). An additional study reported in the journal *Hypertension* found that daily magnesium supplements (480 milligrams) for eight weeks resulted in a small reduction in blood pressure. The effect was most pronounced in subjects with existing high blood pressure and was thought to be due to the fact that magnesium may increase the diameter of blood vessels. You can meet your daily magnesium requirements by eating more seafood, black beans, skim milk, wholegrains, avocados, nuts and dark leafy greens such as spinach.

GET ENOUGH POTASSIUM IN YOUR DIET

Potassium is important for a range of bodily functions. Muscles, including those of the heart, need potassium to contract and beat properly, and potassium is also important in the regulation of blood pressure levels. According to the journal *Circulation*, people with existing high blood pressure levels are less likely than their peers to have a stroke if they consume a diet rich in potassium. A study on nearly 44,000 men found that those with the highest potassium consumption (an intake of about 4.3 grams per day) were 38 per cent less likely to have a stroke than those with the lowest intake (about 2.4 grams per day). Out of interest, this study also found that a high intake of fibre and magnesium reduced the risk of stroke. Potassium is found in high concentrations in fruit, vegetables, plain and unsalted nuts, grains, seeds and legumes. Blood pressure guidelines published in the *Journal of the American Medical Association* also stress the importance of increasing dietary potassium by eating plenty of fruit (such as bananas) and vegetables.

INCLUDE SOME SOY FOODS IN YOUR DIET

The last few decades have seen a rise in the use of soy foods and soy-based products. Soy-based ingredients are cheap to produce and can be added to a wide variety of manufactured food products such as sausages, luncheon meats, protein shakes and bread. Soy foods such as soy milk, soy yoghurt, soy cheese, soy ice-cream and tofu contain isoflavones, which are a class of phytoestrogens. The isoflavones found in soy products have antioxidant properties which can help to keep cholesterol from causing atherosclerotic plaque. Soy foods are also thought to help lower blood cholesterol and reduce the risk of heart disease, although there is mixed research on these benefits. From all the evidence at hand, there seems to be a mild heart health benefit from including some soy products in your diet.

There is also debate about the best type of soy foods to eat. It's thought that unfermented soy foods (soy milk, soy ice-cream) can contain high levels of phytic acid, a substance which can block the absorption of minerals such as calcium, zinc, magnesium and iron. A lot of the soy-based foods consumed in Asian countries are fermented such as tofu, tamari, miso, natto, tempeh and soy sauce. Fermentation of soy foods helps to neutralise the nutrient-depleting phytic acid, potentially making these types of soy food a good choice for your health.

LAUGH MORE

Having a good laugh is no laughing matter when it comes to improving your health. Not only does a good laugh help to relax the muscles in your face, shoulders, neck and upper torso, it also reduces your blood pressure and stress levels. Research conducted at the University of Maryland reported that people who said that they used humour more often were less likely to have had heart attacks. Other research reported to the Society for Neuroscience found that just the anticipation of knowing you will be involved in a positive humorous event days in advance reduces levels of stress hormones in the blood and increases levels of chemicals known to aid relaxation. It also stimulated growth hormone levels by 87 per cent, which is important for the immune system. Some additional health benefits associated with laughter include:

- Laughing can serve as a distraction from worries and lighten stress, anxiety, depression and pain.
- Laughing causes internal exercise, where the lungs inhale and exhale rapidly, improving circulation and oxygen delivery to your vital organs.
- Laughing releases hormones called endorphins that act as natural pain-killers and help to evoke a good mood while lowering the production of stress hormones.
- Laughing releases catecholamines, which have anti-inflammatory properties and improve immune function, which can benefit the heart.

HARNESS THE POWER OF PRAYER

Having religious faith to help deal with everyday stress and life's troubles has been shown to be good for your heart. Stress can be eliminated and/or managed by channelling your energy into more productive endeavours, such as prayers and relaxation. Faith's stress-reducing effects can help alleviate such conditions as high blood pressure and anxiety. A study reported in the journal *Psychosomatic Medicine* found that people with high levels of religious faith had blood pressure readings that were six to seven points lower than their less religious peers. The rhythmic chanting used when saying a prayer of the rosary or performing a yoga mantra seems to have a calming effect on the heart. This tends to slow down your breathing rate, which generally has a positive effect on your cardiovascular and respiratory systems. It seems that getting involved in group activities and cultivating some kind of religious or spiritual faith may promote heart health and boost your wellbeing.

CONSIDER PLANT STEROLS MARGARINES IF OTHER DIETARY CHANGES HAVEN'T WORKED

Plant sterols occur naturally in vegetables, fruits, nuts, grains and seeds, and they are thought to lower blood cholesterol by interfering with the absorption of cholesterol in the gut. By blocking the absorption of cholesterol, less cholesterol is passed into the bloodstream and more cholesterol is excreted when you sit on the toilet. Because plant sterols only occur in small concentrations in nature, food manufacturers have used them as a supplement in some margarines. Research conducted by Australia's CSIRO found that consuming 25 grams of sterol-enriched margarine daily (about the amount you'd use on four slices of bread) helped to lower blood levels of LDL (bad) cholesterol by up to 10 per cent over three weeks.

However, there are a few negatives. The margarine spreads are expensive and they need to be consumed regularly to have a significant effect on reducing blood cholesterol. In other words, you have to keep eating the margarine to maintain the reduction in your cholesterol levels. Large quantities of plant sterols are also thought to reduce the absorption of carotenoids, the antioxidant component of fruits and vegetables that provide protection against oxidation and heart disease.

If your cholesterol levels aren't too high you don't really need to worry about having these spreads. If your cholesterol levels are high, consuming the recommended amount of sterols may be effective. But due to the negative factors I would recommend trying other lifestyle strategies first such as losing excess body fat, eating plenty of fibre and exercising regularly. Finally, if you do resort to using the sterol spreads, make sure you eat plenty of vegetables to compensate for the reduced absorption of antioxidants.

LOWER YOUR LEVEL OF HOMOCYSTEINE

Homocysteine is a substance produced by the body as a by-product of digesting protein. It has an important role to play in the repair and building of body tissue but excessive levels are thought to be an independent risk factor for heart disease and stroke. Homocysteine may increase blood clotting and narrow and harden the blood vessel walls. Approximately 20 to 40 per cent of people who suffer heart disease have elevated levels of homocysteine. However, the link between homocysteine and cardiovascular disease was questioned recently in research published in the *Archives of Internal Medicine*. Future studies will no doubt provide more definitive answers.

In the meantime, it won't do you any harm to try and keep your homocysteine levels down. You can do this by making sure you get enough vitamin B6, B12, folic acid and omega-3 fatty acids in your diet. These vitamins and nutrients help the body break down excessive levels of homocysteine in the liver and allow it to be removed from the bloodstream. It's also wise to avoid large portions of meat and other sources of protein.

Day 41

Know the warning signs of a heart attack and what to do when one occurs

WHAT IS THE IMPACT ON YOUR HEALTH?

A heart attack occurs when the supply of blood to your heart is reduced or blocked and the lack of oxygen can result in irreversible damage to the heart muscle if not evaluated and treated quickly. The impact on your health from a heart attack is immediate and life threatening. Sadly, around one in four heart attacks are fatal. Knowing the symptoms of a heart attack may help to improve your chances of survival or allow you to deliver quick and efficient care for someone else. The symptoms of a heart attack may include:

- Chest pain that ranges from moderate to severe, and lasts for 10 to 15 minutes or longer. It may be described as feeling like a pressure or tightness, burning, squeezing or a crushing sensation.
- The location of chest pain may be in the centre of the chest and may also spread out to the jaw, neck, shoulders and either arm (although it's usually the left). It may also occur in the upper abdomen, where it can be mistaken as an upset stomach.
- Pale appearance, light-headedness, dizziness or fainting.
- There may be an increased heart rate or an irregular beat.
- Weakness, shortness of breath and fatigue on minimal levels of exertion.
- Sweating.
- Nausea and possible vomiting.
- Anxiety.

SCIENCE SAYS

Heart attack does not always cause chest pain — According to the *Annals of Emergency Medicine*, chest pain is a tell-tale sign of a heart attack but it is not the only one. The study of more than 700 patients treated for a heart attack found that nearly half came to the emergency department because of primary symptoms other than chest pain, including shortness of breath, dizziness, weakness or fainting and abdominal pain. According to the researchers, the chances that a person's chief complaint was a symptom other than chest pain increased with age (people older than 84 were least likely to have chest pain). They also reported what has been shown in other studies — that women were more likely than men to have a heart attack without having chest pain.

Gender differences during a heart attack — A study reported in the *Scandinavian Cardiovascular Journal* featuring interviews with over 500 people who had experienced a heart attack found that men and women may experience different types of symptom. Men were more likely than women to report chest symptoms, while women were more likely to complain of nausea, palpitations, shortness of breath, fainting, pain in the back and pain between the shoulder blades. Irrespective of gender, only half the patients thought their symptoms were heart related.

Warning signs one year beforehand — According to research published in the journal *Gender Medicine*, heart attack survivors experienced a number of symptoms within the 12 months leading up to their heart attack. Of the respondents, 62 per cent experienced fatigue, 51 per cent had shoulder or back pain, 45 per cent experienced pain in the chest, 38 per cent experienced arm pain and 33 per cent had shortness of breath. There were no statistically significant gender differences.

Don't wait too long — In a study reported in the journal *Emergency Medicine Australasia*, more than half of the patients who experienced potentially deadly chest pain waited at least 3 hours before going to hospital. This is considered well beyond the time when they can most readily be treated if they are having a heart attack. Sadly, up to 25 per cent of those having a heart attack died within the first hour of symptoms. The researchers recommend that those with chest discomfort should wait no more than 10 minutes before calling an ambulance. The sooner you seek medical attention, the more effective treatment will be.

Know the triggers — According to the journal *Circulation*, heart attack and stroke can be triggered by a variety of stressors, with the most significant being severe emotional stress and heavy physical activity. Lack of sleep, overeating, pollution and cold snaps are also classified as triggers. The researchers found that people can adopt a long-term preventive approach against a specific trigger. For example, regular physical activity reduces the likelihood that a heart attack will be triggered by heavy exertion and stress management techniques can be used to minimise the impact of anger and anxiety.

Heart attacks are more common in the morning — The British Cardiac Patients Association has found that twice as many ambulances are called out for suspected cardiovascular events between 8 a.m. and 10 a.m. compared with any other time of the day. Possible reasons for this include the increased release of adrenaline in the first few hours of the morning or the rise in blood pressure that occurs when people awake from sleep.

Hangover heartache — Research conducted at the University of California found that a severe hangover brought on by binge drinking can increase the risk of having a heart attack. Binge drinking causes dehydration, increases blood pressure and may actually promote clotting after the heavy drinking stops. According to the researchers, this may partially explain why there is a peak in deaths from heart attacks on Mondays.

A warning for sports spectators — According to the *British Medical Journal*, overexcited football fans may be at an increased risk of experiencing a heart attack. The study documented a 50 per cent increase in deaths from heart attack and stroke on the day of an important football match compared with the five days on either side of the game.

PRACTICAL TIPS ON HOW TO DEAL WITH THE SYMPTOMS OF A HEART ATTACK

* Become familiar with the symptoms that people are likely to experience during a heart attack and be aware that there may be a difference between women and men. Unfortunately, it's not uncommon for people to ignore the symptoms, especially when the symptoms seem to go away or are not severe.
* If you are over the age of 65, if you have already had a heart attack or if you have existing signs of heart disease such as diabetes, high cholesterol, high blood pressure, excess body fat or if you are a smoker, pay extra attention

to the signs and symptoms of a heart attack. It's better to err on the side of caution when weighing up a trip to the emergency room.

- The most important factor in surviving a heart attack is seeking out medical attention promptly. Every minute counts when it comes to heart trouble. If you or someone you know is experiencing the symptoms of a heart attack, don't wait longer than 10 minutes to call an ambulance or get someone to hospital. It's estimated that the majority of heart attack patients who are admitted to a hospital survive.
- In many cases a heart attack is triggered by internal electrical disturbances that need to be reversed by a defibrillator — another good reason to stay close to medical attention if you feel the symptoms of a heart attack.
- Some of the reasons people give for not calling for an ambulance earlier include confusion about the symptoms of a heart attack, denial and fearing embarrassment if it's a false alarm. In reality, your life is worth more than a little fear and embarrassment.
- Heart attacks are more common on Mondays and in the morning. Don't wait until the afternoon to go to the emergency department of your nearest hospital or see your GP.
- Consider teaming up with a friend or partner to do a first-aid course that includes training in cardio pulmonary resuscitation (CPR). If the person you spend the most time with knows CPR you can increase each other's chances of survival. If you believe someone is having a heart attack

the following six steps, which encompass the current guidelines for heart resuscitation, can be used as a guide and may help save a life.

1. Remove yourself and the patient from danger.
2. Check for a response (if unresponsive).
3. Call for help.
4. Check for breathing (if not breathing).
5. Give 30 chest compressions (at a rate of almost two compressions per second or 100 per minute).
6. Follow with two quick breaths (stop compressions during breaths) and keep going (alternate the 30 compressions with two breaths) until the ambulance or further help arrives. Brain damage or death may be prevented by mechanically pumping the injured heart.

- Know the difference between a heart attack and heartburn because not all chest pain signals the same thing. Chest pain from indigestion or heartburn has no relation to the heart except for a close proximity of pain. Heartburn is a symptom of reflux, which occurs when gastric acid from the stomach gets into the unprotected esophagus, causing chest pain. While nausea and possible vomiting are also common symptoms, only reflux is likely to cause a bloated feeling after eating, burping, difficulty when swallowing and regurgitation of acid.

- Be aware of the common triggers of a heart attack, especially if you have existing heart disease. Some common triggers include severe emotional stress, heavy physical exertion, binge drinking, cold weather snaps, pollution and roller-coaster rides.

- After calling for an ambulance some experts suggest taking two aspirin if a heart attack seems likely, which is thought to increase blood flow and reduce the risk of death significantly.
- There is a theory (or urban legend) that coughing during a heart attack may help to save your life. However, this technique (cough CPR) is not endorsed by respected organisations such as the American Heart Foundation. It may be used in emergency situations under professional supervision under very specific circumstances but it is not recommended for general use without medical supervision.

Day 42

Have regular heart checks

WHAT IS THE IMPACT ON YOUR HEALTH?

Attending regular check-ups allows you to take control of your heart health and, possibly, your future. The symptoms of heart disease such as high blood pressure or high blood cholesterol can develop without you even knowing it and will often remain undetected for many years. Your risk of heart disease also changes as you age, a fact which underlines the importance of regular, scheduled visits with your doctor. There doesn't need to be something wrong with you to justify a trip to the doctor's — prevention is always better than a cure. Preventive screenings are seen as one of the keys to good health because the earlier diseases are detected, the easier they are to control or cure. Health checks not only alert you to any health problems before they become serious, they also set your mind at ease. Some of the benefits of visiting your doctor regularly for a check-up include:

- Identifying your personal risk factors.
- Identifying which specific actions you need to take to reduce your risk of illness and avoid potential health problems.
- Becoming more aware of the lifestyle habits and behaviours that may lead to future health problems.
- Getting tips and advice on how to improve your health and wellbeing.

Another great benefit of periodic health examinations is that they allow you to develop a better rapport and level of mutual trust with your doctor over time.

SCIENCE SAYS

Know your family health history — According to data presented to the American Society of Human Genetics, family history is a very accurate predictor of disease. Uncovering all the patterns of disease that lurk in your family tree is important and holiday gatherings are a good opportunity to gather information.

Siblings' heart problems the best predictor for you A research finding published in the journal *Circulation*, is that your brother or sister is a better predictor of heart disease than your parents. The study of nearly 8500 adults discovered that people were 2.5 times more likely to have coronary atherosclerosis (heart and artery disease) if a brother or sister had already been diagnosed with heart disease. The researchers maintain that this is important to know because most people ask their parents for their health history and overlook their siblings.

Simple heart checks could save lives — According to the Royal College of Physicians in the United Kingdom, hundreds of thousands of people are at risk from an undiagnosed heart condition. The researchers found that early detection allows for lifestyle changes that can reduce risk, prevent disease and improve life expectancy to normal.

Many don't know their numbers — A survey of 1000 people conducted by *Prevention* magazine found that 70 per cent of respondents didn't know what their blood cholesterol was. In addition, around 75 per cent of respondents didn't know the difference between good (HDL) and bad (LDL) cholesterol.

Check-up advised after family tragedy — Recommendations published in the *Journal of the American College of Cardiology*, advocate that anyone with a close relative who suffered a sudden cardiac death should make it a priority to see their doctor.

Earlier testing for heart disease encouraged — Research reported in the *Journal of the American Medical Association* suggests that the risk of heart disease can be identified early in life and that cholesterol and other tests should be initiated earlier than they now are. According to the researchers, children and adolescents with several risk factors are at an increased risk of developing atherosclerosis in adulthood. They also believe that reductions in risk could potentially be achieved in children by introducing lifestyle modifications such as dietary changes, increased levels of physical activity and control of obesity.

PRACTICAL TIPS ON SCHEDULING REGULAR HEALTH CHECKS

- Before visiting your doctor it is helpful to investigate the medical history of your mother, father, sisters and brothers. This helps your doctor to determine the diseases from which you are most at risk and which precautionary tests are necessary. Your family's health history can also be helpful in identifying risk factors that can be managed with lifestyle changes. You can minimise the risk or even overcome some inherited tendencies if you have a healthy diet and an active lifestyle.
- Book an appointment with your doctor and don't be afraid to write down any symptoms, changes, concerns and questions in preparation for the visit. Also, be prepared to be open and honest about your lifestyle, informing your doctor about any other treatments or therapies that you are using, including natural therapies, diet, exercise programs and stress management techniques.
- Some typical questions you may want to ask your doctor include how much physical activity should I be doing, am I due for any health tests, what diet should I follow to address my personal risk factors and is there anything new

in lifestyle strategies you've been made aware of since my last visit?

- The following table is a guide as to how often you should schedule particular health checks relevant to your heart health. However, some medical professionals disagree about how often people should be tested, so discuss with your doctor what frequency is best for you and your circumstances.

Health checks	In your 20s and 30s	In your 40s and 50s	When you're 60 and older
Blood pressure	Every two years	Every year	Every year
Cholesterol	Once at 30, then every five years. Every two years if there is a family history.	Every five years, or every two if there is a family history.	Every two years, or every year if you have had a problem in the past.
Blood glucose test	Every year if you have a family history of diabetes.	Every year if you have a family history of diabetes, or if you are obese.	Every two years. Every year if you have a family history of diabetes, if you are obese, or if you have high blood pressure.
Waist (at navel)	Every year	Every year	Every year

- If your doctor suspects any irregularities, they may seek to do more extensive testing. This may involve an electrocardiogram (ECG), a chest X-ray, an exercise stress test, a CT scan or a cardiac catheterisation.
- Research has shown that men use health services less frequently than women do even though they are at a higher risk of suffering heart disease. And it's not just regular check-ups that men avoid; they also shy away from seeking

out a doctor when they are really sick. Issues such as fear, denial, embarrassment and threatened masculinity are all reasons why men may not want to go to the doctor. Some men may be more willing if certain family members are present. Men who realise the importance of preventative health care can help to save themselves from much worse pain and embarrassment down the track.

- A health check for heart disease is just as important for women. Although women are less likely to get heart disease than men, a higher percentage of women diagnosed with heart disease will die from it.

Can I continue to inform and motivate you?

Why not subscribe to my free newsletter

I am genuinely passionate about health, fitness and wellness, and I am driven to help people enjoy the benefits it has to offer. I also love to keep people informed on the latest in health and wellness. The *Better Body Update* is a free weekly email newsletter that includes information on fat loss, fitness, nutrition, heart health and motivation, with occasional success stories from other people who have achieved their health and fitness goals. You'll also find a motivational quote to help inspire you and keep you on track. It's only short, it's completely free and you can subscribe by visiting my website. You can also unsubscribe at any time. I guarantee that your personal details will remain personal.

While you're at my website you can download sample

chapters from my previous books and read some of the weight-loss articles I've had published. You can also find out more about my online personal training and weight-loss coaching. If you'd like to know more about my freelance writing and public speaking services, please contact me.

If you have any questions, queries or concerns about your health or the information in this book, please don't hesitate to contact me. If you have a positive experience you'd like to share after following the strategies in this book, I'd love to hear from you too. I'll do my best to get back to you as soon as possible.

email: info@andrewcate.com
website: www.andrewcate.com
postal address: Andrew Cate
                  13A Waterview Street
                  Mona Vale, NSW, 2103
                  Australia

www.ingramcontent.com/pod-product-compliance
Lightning Source LLC
Chambersburg PA
CBHW032129020426
42334CB00016B/1089